Vaccines and Informed Choice

everything parents need to know

6th Edition

by

Patty Brennan

© 1995 Patty Brennan
2nd Edition, 1998
3rd Edition, 2004
4th Edition, 2009
5th Edition, 2014
6th Edition, 2015

Published in the United States by
Dream Street Press
Ann Arbor, Michigan

ISBN-13: 978-1512064094
ISBN-10: 1512064092

Disclaimer
The content of this book is for informational and educational purposes only. The information is not intended to replace professional medical evaluation or advice. The author is not responsible for and will not be liable for any direct, indirect, consequential, special, exemplary or other damages arising from the use or misuse of any information presented. For those who want the homeopathic alternative, please seek care from a qualified "classical homeopath."

The decision whether or not to vaccinate is a personal one. The author is not a health care practitioner nor legal advisor and makes no claim in this regard. Nor does the author recommend for or against vaccines. The information in this book is compiled from other sources. If you have questions or doubts about any material presented, please check the documented sources.

Primum non nocere . . .

First, not to harm

—Hippocrates

ACKNOWLEDGMENTS

I'd like to acknowledge the valuable contributions of my husband, Gerald Brennan, whose enthusiastic support of all my endeavors is much appreciated. Thanks are also due to author/publisher Jane Sheppard for granting permission to reprint two articles, *Antibiotics: How Do They Harm Our Children?* and *Strengthening a Weakened Immune System.*

CONTENTS

Acknowledgments

Preface – 1

Options for Parents – 5

The Case against Compulsory Vaccination – 9
      The Government and Vaccine Safety
      The Vaccine Mandate Process
      Are Vaccines Effective?
      The Concept and Ethics of Herd Immunity
      How the Immune System Works
      How Vaccinations Work

Vaccine Overview – 23
      Diphtheria (DTaP)
      Haemophilus Influenza Type B (HIB)
      Hepatitis A
      Hepatitis B
      Human Papillomavirus (HPV)
      Influenza
      Measles (MMR)
      Meningococcal
      Mumps (MMR)
      Pertussis (Whooping Cough) (DTaP)
      Pneumoccal (Pn)
      Polio (IP for "inactivated Polio")
      Rotavirus
      Rubella (MMR)
      Tetanus (DTaP)
      Varicella Zoster (Chicken Pox)

Adverse Reactions to Vaccinations – 51
Vaccine Ingredients
Vaccine Risks
Preventing Vaccine Reactions
Legal Recourse for Adverse Vaccine Reactions

Enhancing the Immune System Naturally – 63
Do Germs Cause Disease?
Understanding Disease Symptoms
Building the Immune System
A Special Note on Fevers
Antibiotics: How Do They Harm Our Children?
Food and Herbal Sources of Important Immune
    System Nutrients
Family Winter Health Tea Recipe
Stimulating a Weakened Immune System

The Role of Homeopathy – 85
Introduction to Homeopathy
Homeopathy and Vaccine Reactions
Homeopathic Prophylaxis and Treatment of
    Infectious Childhood Diseases
Homeopathic "Vaccines"

Claiming an Exemption – 103
When are Waivers Required?
General Recommendations
Medical Exemptions
Religious Exemptions
Philosophical/Other Exemptions
Strategies/Considerations
Exceptions/Limitations on Exemptions
If Your Exemption is Denied
Dealing with Coercion

Vigilance is the Price of Freedom
Finding a Doctor Who Supports Parental Choice

In Conclusion – 113

Resources – 115
Vaccine Controversies
Natural Approaches to Developing the Immune
System
Homeopathy
World Travel

About the Author – 123

PREFACE

Who is the intended reader of this book?

I have been a consumer-oriented childbirth educator since 1983. In that work, my focus has been to acquaint expectant parents with the choices before them and to present them with the benefits and risks inherent in each choice, as well as available alternatives. I am dedicated to the concept that parents should learn to ask the right questions and then make informed choices.

This book is not a primary source of information on the vaccine issue, but rather a distillation of the heavily-documented work of others. When I first began to research the subject of vaccines from the perspective of a parent and consumer health safety advocate, I found a daunting amount of information to sort through. I identified a need for this information to be condensed and synthesized so that it could be presented to parents as "these are the questions you should be asking about vaccination." The following areas of focus emerged: (1) controversies—vaccine efficacy, benefits and risks; (2) prevention of adverse vaccine reactions; (3) enhancing natural immunity; (4) the role of homeopathy; and (5) vaccine politics (or how government vaccine policy is made and the protection of parental rights). This book is organized around these themes. For readers seeking detailed primary sources of information summarized here, please go directly to the authors cited.

My Journey

In 1980, I took a healthy child to the doctor's office and I brought home a sick baby. For the week following administration of the MMR vaccine, my son ran a high fever, could not sit to drink, stopped walking and was lethargic. I remember running to the grocery store in a panic for a baby bottle because he could not manage drinking from a straw and I was no longer breastfeeding. My son recovered, having suffered what was deemed to be a "moderate" systemic vaccine reaction. But I was changed. I kept thinking, "What's wrong with this picture?" The seed had been planted for my path as a consumer health advocate and educator.

Thirty-five years later, as an increasing number of new vaccines are added to the recommended schedules, I remain concerned if not alarmed. Children today receive 69 doses of vaccines for 16 different viral and bacterial illnesses. This more than doubles the government childhood schedule of 34 doses of 11 different vaccines in the year 2000. Question: Is there evidence that U.S. children today are healthier?

As I have followed the vaccination controversy closely over the years, I have come to the conclusion that anyone who seriously examines the issue is likely to become skeptical and have reservations about wholeheartedly embracing all vaccines. Such is my bias. That said, I did not set out to write an anti-vaccine diatribe. I do not believe that there is one right approach or path for every family, nor do I presume to know what is best for you, the reader, and your children and grandchildren. I simply want to encourage you to ask questions. I want you to know your rights and understand your full range of options. And further, if vaccination does seem to you to be the best pathway for optimizing your children's health, that it be undertaken in a way that minimizes the risk of adverse reactions.

This book grew out of a series of lectures given throughout the past three-plus decades and first published under the title *Vaccine Choices, Homeopathic Alternatives & Parental Rights* in 1995. The material in the 6th Edition has been substantially updated with the most recent information available on the topic. In the case of those who are looking for pro-vaccination arguments, you will not find what you seek here. My position is that pro-vaccine ideology is prevalent in our culture. One does not need to seek it out. What is largely missing, in my view, is accessible information on the other side of the issue and I have attempted to fill that gap here.

My Sources

Neil Miller of the Think Twice Global Vaccine Institute [http:/www.thinktwice.com] is the author of a number of books on vaccines in which he reports meticulously researched epidemiological public health data on vaccine efficacy and safety. His works are heavily referenced here (see Resources).

Dr. Sherri Tenpenny offers an in-depth examination of the risks associated with vaccines in her two DVD presentations, *Vaccines—The Risks, Benefits and Choices* and *Vaccines: What CDC Documents and Science Reveal.* Dr. Tenpenny has sorted through abstracts and citations from CDC documents and respected peer-reviewed medical journals. She shares information that establishes links between vaccines and allergies, asthma, seizures and neurological disorders in children and offers highly-documented proof that vaccines can compromise the immune system. [http:/www.drtenpenny.com]

Dr. Robert W. Sears is a pro-vaccine advocate and author of *The Vaccine Book: Making the Right Decision for Your Child,* 2nd Edition (2011). For parents who choose to vaccinate, this book serves as a guide to the least toxic vaccines on the market and provides an alternate vaccine schedule designed to limit toxic exposure. I cannot wholeheartedly recommend the book as there are problems with Dr. Sears' essentially pro-vaccine, pro-herd-immunity viewpoint. He unquestioningly embraces the notion that vaccines have the potential to completely eradicate the diseases they are designed to prevent and that public health policy towards this end is desirable (the more the better, apparently). There is a presumption of trust in the vaccine industry and government policy makers which history has demonstrated is unwarranted. With a sarcastic dismissal, Sears refuses to give any credence to the notion that germs may not be the *cause* of disease, while alternative approaches to the prevention and treatment of disease are altogether ignored.
Nevertheless, Sears upholds parents' right to choose and for this he should be applauded.

OPTIONS FOR PARENTS

In spite of pervasive efforts to promote compliance with recommended vaccination programs by the pharmaceutical industry, the U.S. government, the American Medical Association (AMA), the American Academy of Pediatricians (AAP), and the mainstream media, concerns regarding vaccine safety continue to emerge. This book is designed to help parents become better informed consumers of health care by encouraging them to obtain *informed consent* to vaccinations *or* to exercise their (often not recognized) *right to informed refusal* of vaccines. Informed parents have the following choices before them:

- *Go with the program*: Make educated decisions regarding vaccine brands and timing options and take precautions to prevent bad reactions; know your treatment options if your child experiences a bad reaction; know your rights.
- *Flexible program*: Choose some vaccines and decline others; or choose an alternate timetable, perhaps delaying some vaccines until your child is older (with a more developed immune system) and actually facing higher risk of exposure or danger from exposure (e.g., hepatitis B, HPV, tetanus, rubella); make educated decisions regarding vaccine brands; give vaccines one at a time; take precautions to prevent bad reactions; know your treatment options if your child experiences a bad reaction; know your rights.

- *Refuse all vaccines*: Use homeopathy or other non-toxic methods of preventing and treating disease; know your rights.

Informed consent to vaccination involves knowing the answers to the following questions for each vaccine:

- What is the seriousness of the diseases to be immunized against?
- What is the risk of an epidemic in my area?
- How effective is the vaccine in preventing disease?
- How safe is the vaccine?
- Are some brands of the vaccine safer than others and which brand does my doctor give?
- Does my child have any contraindications for this vaccine?
- How can I protect my child from adverse reactions to vaccines?
- Is there any way to protect my child without vaccinating? What are the alternatives?
- What are my legal rights regarding "mandatory" vaccines?

An additional step that parents can take, regardless of their choice, is to do all that is within their power to build their child's immune system and to have treatment options and resources in place in the event that their child becomes ill. Vaccines or no vaccines, this seems prudent. In this book, the homeopathic alternative is emphasized, but the contributions of breastfeeding, nutrition, herbs, chiropractic care and more are encouraged.

So, what is "the program"? See below for current recommendations of the AAP. Please note, however, that not all of these vaccines are currently "mandated" in every state, though some physicians may recommend them. Vaccines that may not be required in all states include influenza, hepatitis A, HPV, meningococcal, PCV and rotavirus. This information should be available on your state's website.

Birth	HepB
1 month	HepB
2 months	RV, DTaP, Hib, PCV, IPV
4 months	RV, DTaP, Hib, PCV, IPV
6 months	HepB, RV, DTaP, Hib, PCV, IPV,
Influenza	annual
1 year	Hib, PCV, MMR, Varicella, HepA
15 months	DTaP
4–6 years	DTaP, IPV, MMR, Varicella
11–12 years	DTaP, Meningococcal, HPV (3 doses)

DTaP = diphtheria, tetanus, acellular pertussis
HepA = hepatitis A
HepB = hepatitis B
Hib = haemophilus influenza type B
HPV = human papilloma virus
IPV = inactivated polio virus
MMR = measles, mumps, rubella
PCV = pneumococcal
RV = rotovirus
Varicella = chickenpox

Source:
[http://www.cdc.gov/vaccines/schedules/downloads/child/0-18yrs-schedule.pdf]

THE CASE AGAINST COMPULSORY VACCINATION

The Government and Vaccine Safety

Vaccinating your child against infectious diseases may not always be a matter of choice. In state legislatures across the nation, new laws designed to limit parents' right to choose in this important health matter are regularly introduced. An increasing number of states are enacting legislation to eliminate religious and philosophical exemptions. Parents who are non-compliant with vaccine mandates may become increasingly vulnerable to charges of "medical neglect," thereby providing grounds for the Department of Children's Protective Services (CPS) to remove children from a parent's care.

In 1993, Senator Ted Kennedy proposed that a computerized federal tracking system be developed for all U.S. children (from birth onwards, through their social security numbers) to ensure the means to enforce such laws. Subsequently, after President Clinton's efforts to implement a federal monitoring system failed to pass Congress, the Centers for Disease Control (CDC) began to incentivize states and major cities to develop their own tracking systems. In 2010, the Patient Protection and Affordable Care Act passed into law. This law, among other things, incentivizes doctors to convert patient data into electronic health record formats that can be shared across state and federal electronic databases, thereby enabling the tracking of national vaccine coverage rates, while identifying who is and is not vaccinated. Though many states already have vaccine tracking registries (Immunization Information

Systems) in place, current law prevents sharing of personal medical information. Thus, financial and other types of incentives are being implemented to convince vaccine providers and state legislators to participate in the gathering of this private medical information on all Americans. It is not paranoid, nor does it take a great leap of imagination to see the direction the government is heading.

Under the current tracking systems, parents are issued reminders and vaccination status of a child will most assuredly be checked anytime that child interfaces with the medical system—such as a visit to a pediatrician's office, urgent care or hospital emergency room—and coercive pressure brought to bear at a vulnerable time. The combination of an injured child and vaccine non-compliance constitutes a red flag whereby CPS may be notified by ER personnel.

Because of the impending specter of compulsory vaccination, U.S. citizens are entitled to proof beyond a reasonable doubt that mass vaccination schemes are a *safe and effective* means of preventing infectious diseases. Investigation shows clearly that such evidence does not exist. In 2000, the Congressional Committee on Government Reform, chaired by Congressman Dan Burton (R–Indiana), initiated an investigation into federal vaccine policy focusing on issues regarding vaccine safety and research. One area of investigation centered on conflict of interest on the part of federal policy makers. It was discovered that many individuals serving on two key advisory committees—the Food & Drug Administration's (FDA) Vaccines and Related Biological Products Advisory Committee (VRBPAC) and the CDC's Advisory Committee on Immunizations Practices (ACIP)—had substantial financial ties to pharmaceutical companies that manufacture vaccines under consideration by the committees. In a review of the rotavirus vaccine approval process, for example, three out of five members on the FDA licensing committee that approved the vaccine were found to have a conflict of interest. See my discussion on page 43 regarding the rotavirus vaccine fiasco and you will understand why this finding should give us all pause.

In a letter to the Department of Health and Human Services (DHHS) Secretary Shalala, Congressman Burton summarized as follows:

> *"For the public to have confidence in the decisions made by their government, they must be assured that those decisions are not being affected by conflict of interest. It has become clear over the course of this investigation that the VRBPAC and the ACIP are dominated by individuals with close working relationships with the vaccine producers. This was never the intent of the Federal Advisory Committee Act, which requires that a diversity of views be represented on advisory committees."*

It was through Congressman Burton's efforts, that *most* (though not all) of the neurotoxin mercury has been removed from childhood vaccines. It is worth noting that Burton's interest in the vaccine controversy is due to the fact that he has two grandchildren who were both developmentally normal prior to receiving the MMR (measles, mumps, rubella) vaccine, but became autistic soon after the vaccine was administered.

Recent work by Dr. Sherri Tenpenny (see Resources) on vaccine safety also raises concerns. Both

Dr. Tenpenny and Dr. Sears address the issue of inadequate long-term safety research prior to FDA licensing of new vaccines. *There is a presumption of benefit given to all vaccines.* This can be contrasted with the FDA approach to other new pharmaceuticals which must go through years of trials in a select group of people, compared to a control group, to ensure safety. Vaccines, on the other hand, do not follow the double-blind "gold standard" of research. The control group for vaccines is to compare the safety profile of vaccine test recipients against a known vaccine's safety profile or compare populations of countries that use a vaccine and those that don't. According to Sears, "virtually every product insert states that the vaccine was tested alongside existing vaccines, not in isolation." Yet another drawback of existing "safety studies" is that they include only healthy children, even though all children are given a vaccine once the trials are over (including sick children who show up with a fever in the ER).

One justification for this approach is that, because of the presumption of benefit given to all vaccines, it is considered unethical to withhold vaccination from a control group. Author Trevor Gunn (see Resources) summarizes this key point:

> *"While it is said to be unethical to leave one group 'unprotected' to create the placebo group from which to do the comparisons, note that almost all other drugs are required to undergo this procedure. Clearly the supposition is that the advantage of the vaccine must outweigh any disadvantage; the presupposition is that the vaccine works, then logically it would be*

unethical to create a non-vaccinated (placebo) group. This is of course a circular argument, the point of the trial would be to determine that very premise; you cannot know that a vaccine benefit outweighs any disadvantage over and above natural immunity until you carry out such a trial.... [However], it is very difficult to question core beliefs, especially when our incomes are tied to the continuation of those core beliefs and associated practices."

Consider also that "safety studies" are undertaken by the vaccine manufacturers themselves rather than via independent oversight agencies. For example, a much-publicized study that concluded there was no link between the MMR vaccine and the development of autism was done by a manufacturer of the MMR vaccine. Since greed, corruption and conflict of interest have been demonstrated, each consumer needs to decide just how comfortable he/she is with the level of safety testing that is done as more and more new vaccines receive approval. Essentially, our children become the true test subjects when new vaccines are introduced. Are you comfortable with this?

The pharmaceutical companies comprise a powerful political lobby in the U.S. The government has already freed them from liability concerns vis-à-vis vaccines, so that the taxpayer picks up the bill when a vaccine can be proven to cause damage to an individual (a difficult case to make, especially in the instance of long-term effects on health). What other industry has a government-mandated assurance that their products will be purchased? There is a tremendous profit to be made with the production and approval of each new vaccine, providing incentive to get new vaccines to the market quickly. Today, American children are being told by government health officials and pediatricians to get 69 doses of 16 vaccines between birth and age 18. In 2015, the vaccine industry is expected to sell approximately $24 billion worth of vaccines.

Given that (1) one in two Americans suffers from chronic disease, (2) America ranks 26th in infant mortality and (3) 25 percent of U.S. children are suffering from learning disabilities, ADHD, severe allergies, autism, asthma, diabetes, inflammatory bowel disorder, rheumatoid arthritis and other chronic immune and brain disorders, it seems logical to ask, along with Barbara Loe Fisher of the National Vaccine Information Center (NVIC), "Why is the most highly vaccinated child population in the world so sick and disabled?"

The Vaccine Mandate Process

First comes approval, followed by recommendations for use, and finally, government mandates. When vaccines fail to provide adequate protection from disease over time, the schedule gets changed and "booster" shots are recommended. That is the process. The reverse process, once a mandated vaccine is determined to be dangerous, is inexplicably more cumbersome and, in the case of the rotavirus, DPT and oral polio vaccines, many children suffered harm, even after problems with the vaccine were reported.

Following is a list of steps to vaccine licensing and government mandates:

(1) Drug manufacturer applies to the FDA to start clinical trials of a new vaccine.

(2) Drug company conducts three phases of clinical trials that do *not* involve double-blind testing of research subjects.

(3) The VRBPAC reviews and evaluates data on the clinical trials supplied by the drug company and then advises the FDA on licensing of the vaccine for commercial use.

(4) Following recommendation by the VRBPAC, the FDA grants a license to manufacture the vaccine.

(5) The ACIP advises the CDC on guidelines to be issued to doctors and the states for the appropriate use of vaccines. Vaccine policy guidelines include recommended routine administration for pediatric and adult populations, schedules regarding the appropriate periodicity and dosage, and contraindications applicable to vaccines. According to Barbara Loe Fisher of the NVIC, "the recommendation for routine use of a vaccine by this committee is tantamount to a federal mandate" [http://www.909shot.com/COFRpt.htm].

(6) Recommendations by the ACIP become official after approval by the Director of the CDC and the Secretary of the Department of Health and Human Services (DHHS), and publication in the *Morbidity and Mortality Weekly Report (MMWR)*.

(7) State legislatures then pass laws to mandate use of selected vaccines.

(8) The government relies upon the Vaccine
Adverse Event Reporting System (VAERS) to
identify problems with the vaccine after
marketing begins.

Are Vaccines Effective?

Investigation of disease incidence rates shows that the
acute infectious diseases for which vaccines have been
developed have enjoyed a steep decline over time. In
some cases, declines occurred prior to introduction of
the vaccine. In others, researchers question whether or
not the related vaccine is actually responsible for the
decline.

Even superficial investigation suggests that
infectious diseases have their own natural history and
limited lifespan quite independent of mankind's
attempts to eradicate them. The implementation of
quarantines and improved hygiene and living conditions
coincided with a drastic falling off in the number of
cases of pertussis, diphtheria, tetanus, cholera, typhoid
and tuberculosis long before vaccinations were
developed for them. See also our discussion of Measles
on page 32. For further detailed analysis on this subject,
I refer you to the work of Dr. Neil Miller, in particular
Are Vaccines Safe and Effective? Dr. Miller directly
analyzes public health data on disease incidence.

Another researcher, Dr. Sherri Tenpenny, begins
her discussion on vaccines with the following
definitions:

> *"Vaccination* is the physical act of administering a
> vaccine or toxoid. *Immunization* is the process of

inducing artificial immunity by introducing an immunobiologic."

Dr. Tenpenny emphasizes that the two terms are not synonymous. A shot does not equal immunity, nor does it necessarily mean that the recipient has the antibody. Furthermore, antibody production does not equal protection. To say that vaccines are effective means that they have the power to induce the intended results. Dr. Tenpenny distinguishes between "research efficacy" (the ability to evoke antibody response) and "clinical efficacy" (the ability to prevent infections) and states that vaccine science is based on research efficacy, not clinical efficacy. She cites chickenpox, pertussis and HIB manufacturer's statements to the effect that a direct correlation between antibody response and protection against the disease has not been demonstrated or is "unknown."

The Concept and Ethics of Herd Immunity
Epidemiologists who study disease patterns and outbreaks have concluded that when a certain percentage of a given population has immunity to a specific disease, then epidemics do not develop. The folks who have immunity, therefore, provide protection against the disease to those who do not. The exact percentage level needed to provide "herd immunity" for a given disease is not known. In the case of measles, for example, target rates from 67 to 100 percent are quoted in the literature (Miller, *Vaccines, Autism, and Childhood Disorders*).

In a discussion of herd immunity for rubella, Miller summarizes the following concern:

"Research has shown that most persons who contract rubella as adults do so through contact with other adults. Since children are not the primary 'herd' infecting pregnant women, some authorities argue, they should not be targeted for vaccination. Is it ethical for one herd—children—to be force-inoculated, denied natural immunity, and subjected to all of the potential side-effects, so that another herd—the unborn fetuses of rubella-susceptible pregnant women—may theoretically be protected?"

Pro-vaccine advocates criticize parents who choose not to vaccinate, alleging that the unvaccinated children benefit from the vaccinated status of others. Advocates further theorize that if a growing number of parents refuse vaccines, herd immunity will be lost and we will see a corresponding resurgence of deadly diseases. The implication is that such a choice shows reckless disregard for public health on the part of the unvaccinated.

My position is that, in the end, each parent must decide whether evidence supports the theory that vaccines enhance health or not and to undertake our own benefit versus risk analysis for each vaccine. Blind trust in a flawed system is not due diligence. If we endeavor to make an informed decision, then, at the very least, we will not be subjecting our children to unnecessary risk for unproven benefit.

How the Immune System Works
Let's consider a normal course of measles. It's generally agreed that a susceptible person inhales the virus from

contact with the air around a coughing or sneezing person who already has the disease. Once inside the respiratory system, the virus multiplies wildly. The first tissues to be infected are the tonsils, adenoids and associated structures. Then the lymph nodes inflame and the virus passes into the bloodstream and enters the spleen, thymus, liver and bone marrow.

Throughout this initial phase of infection the patient is largely unaware of any problems, though this is the most contagious stage of the disease. By the time a couple of weeks have passed, the first symptoms appear as the body mounts its counter-attack, circulating the appropriate antibodies as a small part of the total immune system response. A fever lasting 3–4 days is the first symptom, followed by the rash. *The symptoms peak at the same time as the antibody response.* This indicates that what is experienced as the misery of a measles infection is, in fact, the effort of the immune system to clear the measles virus from the body. The measles rash is the final stage of elimination of the virus through the skin.

The acute illness is an opportunity for the immune system to develop strength and resistance. Once the body defeats the virus, it is forever immune to the illness. In fact, experiencing measles is the only way to gain true and lasting immunity to the disease. It is also the only way that a mother can pass immune factors on to her babies to protect them in the early vulnerable months of life. Interestingly, practitioners of Traditional Chinese Medicine contend that measles presents an opportunity for the child to eliminate poisons accumulated while in the womb. Overall, Western medicine does not embrace the notion that illness can be purposeful, a concept that is prevalent in holistic systems.

How Vaccinations Work

There are four main types of vaccines:

- polysaccharide conjugate vaccines—do not contain the entire germ; one cannot become infected with the disease from the vaccine
- live-viral vaccines—contain the whole living virus; in rare instances, recipient can become infected with the disease
- killed-viral vaccines—contain the whole germ, but it has been killed so it cannot infect the recipient
- recombinant vaccine—genetically engineered and does not contain any portion of the original germ, though it does have some manufactured proteins that match the germ's proteins

The primary aim of all types of vaccines is to stimulate the production of blood antibodies for a specific disease-causing pathogen, which will remain in the body to recognize and protect against future contact with that pathogen.

By injecting an individual with the attenuated live-virus measles vaccine, all of the body's natural ports-of-entry are bypassed and the virus is placed directly into the bloodstream. The virus has been attenuated (or altered) so that it will not produce the generalized inflammatory response that signals the healthy body's reaction to the invading microbes. This means that there is no all-out attack to remove the offending organisms.

Instead, the body substitutes a low-level chronic condition for the natural acute response. The virus remains in the body for a long time, perhaps permanently, while a constant low-level struggle is being waged by the immune system. This is why vaccines are capable of preventing acute cases of the diseases that they are designed to thwart. Instead of providing true immunity, vaccines initiate a chronic and low-level case of the illness. This may result in a progressively weakened response from the immune system to the disease state. Technically, vaccines do not confer true immunity.

Long-term adverse effects on the immune system have been written about by many researchers. It's been long understood that live viruses are capable of surviving in their host's body for many years without provoking an acute disease reaction. As the latent virus fuses its genetic code to the cell which it infests, it replicates along with the infected cells. Eventually, what the body considers its self can become confused with what the body considers an invader, and the immune system now finds that it must attack the cells themselves. These latent viruses have been implicated as factors predisposing people to a variety of chronic conditions including auto-immune disorders such as Chronic Fatigue Syndrome, AIDS and cancer.

In his booklet, *The Case Against Immunization* (see Resources), Dr. Moskowitz suggests that the result of using vaccines to control disease "is essentially to trade off our acute epidemic diseases of the past century for the far less curable chronic diseases of the present." A growing body of evidence (see Sears) demonstrates that Moskowitz's concerns are well founded. Is it a coincidence that we are seeing an increase in chronic disease as the number of vaccines given in early childhood is on the rise? It seems a question worth investigating.

VACCINE OVERVIEW

The vaccines discussed below are not all mandated in every state. However, they may be recommended or pushed by your pediatrician or other medical personnel with whom you have contact.

Diphtheria (DTaP)

<u>Agent</u>: a bacterial infection of the upper respiratory tract.

<u>Disease Symptoms</u>: fever, sore throat, swollen cervical glands; a thick, gelatinous membrane develops on the tonsils and throat and may descend into the windpipe and lungs making breathing and swallowing dangerously difficult; complications include inflammation of the heart muscle, paralysis of the throat, eye and respiratory muscles, which can be fatal.

<u>Vaccine History & Effectiveness</u>: Widespread immunization began in the early 1940s. Diphtheria vaccine is given today as one component of the DTaP. It is an inactivated bacterial vaccine made from toxins produced by the diphtheria bacterium (or *toxoid)* and then rendered harmless by a chemical agent (usually formaldehyde). Between 1900 and 1930, before the vaccine was introduced, the U.S. had already seen a decline in diphtheria death rates of more than 90 percent. Since World War II, in every country where the vaccine was introduced, the number of diphtheria cases soared dramatically. The FDA was obliged to report in 1975 that the diphtheria vaccine "is not as effective an immunization agent as might be anticipated." Today,

diphtheria is very rare in the U.S. with less than five confirmed cases per year.

Vaccine Risks: Adverse reactions include vomiting, anorexia, convulsions and various allergic reactions severe enough to cause death.

Haemophilus Influenza Type B (HIB)

Agent: bacterial infection causing inflammation of the membranes of the spinal cord or brain.

Disease Symptoms: fever, headache, intolerance to light and sound; delirium, convulsions, coma; can be life-threatening; long-term complications include hearing loss and learning disabilities. HIB has been suspected of involvement not only in the deadly meningitis, but also in upper respiratory and ear infections, inflamed sinuses and pneumonia. Peak incidence of the disease is between 6 and 7 months of age. Fifty percent of all cases are in children less than one year old. Children under six months of age are protected by maternal antibodies and breastfeeding is known to reduce incidence rates. Large daycare settings pose an increased risk, by as much as 50 percent. Conversely, a breastfed child who is at home until the age of 18 months is at low risk for the disease. Meningitis is extremely rare (approximately 25 cases per year in the U.S. in kids under age five).

Vaccine History & Effectiveness: The HIB vaccine is a new-generation vaccine, approved for use in 1985. In a preliminary CDC study, the first HIB vaccine showed an efficacy rate of only 41 percent. Other studies vary widely in their results, with one study reporting that HIB-vaccinated children in Minnesota were found to be five times *more likely* to contract meningitis in the first week following vaccination, than non-vaccinated children. This vaccine is mandated in some states only for children entering pre-school childcare programs.

Vaccine Risks: Reactions include fever, pain and swelling at the injection site, rash, hives, irritability, restless sleep, prolonged crying, diarrhea, vomiting, loss of appetite, convulsions and collapse; suspected link with the development of juvenile-onset diabetes.

Hepatitis A

Agent: a virus that attacks the liver, causing temporary liver inflammation; contamination passed from stool to mouth. Increased risk in daycare settings, beaches contaminated with sewage runoff and developing countries with poor hygiene. In the U.S., hepatitis A is primarily found in the following states: Arizona, Alaska, Oregon, New Mexico, Utah, Washington, Oklahoma, South Dakota, Idaho, Nevada and California.

Disease Symptoms: mild in children; fairly severe in teens and adults; intestinal influenza symptoms that can last for a few weeks; jaundice; people with underlying liver disease can suffer severe liver damage from hepatitis A; most others recover in a few weeks with no ill effects.

Vaccine History & Effectiveness: Available since the mid-1980s, the vaccine was only recommended for children two years and older who were living in a high-risk area of the country, but as of 2006, it has been recommended for all children nationwide.

Vaccine Risks: More common reports of standard side effects, seizures (higher incidence if given before age two), Guillain-Barre syndrome, encephalitis, encephalopathy, nerve problems and multiple sclerosis.

Guillain-Barre is mentioned frequently as a risk for many vaccines. Guillain-Barre syndrome is a disorder in which the body's immune system attacks part of the peripheral nervous system. The first symptoms of this disorder include varying degrees of weakness or tingling sensations in the legs. In many instances the weakness and abnormal sensations spread to the arms and upper body. These symptoms can increase in intensity until certain muscles cannot be used at all and, when severe, the patient is almost totally paralyzed. Most patients recover from even the most severe form of the disease, although some continue to experience weakness and it is associated with chronic fatigue syndrome.

Hepatitis B

Agent: virus which attacks the liver and is found in body fluids of infected persons.

Disease Symptoms: early symptoms include nausea, vomiting, fatigue, loss of appetite, changes in smelling and taste, rash, joint pain, headache, cough; more advanced symptoms include dark urine, clay-colored stools and jaundice; the liver can become enlarged and tender with pain in the upper right abdomen. Most people who have the disease do not need to be hospitalized and 90 percent recover completely. Rare complications include severe brain inflammation, gastrointestinal bleeding, respiratory and cardiac collapse, renal and liver failure, coma and death. There are suspected links with the development of multiple sclerosis and rheumatoid arthritis.

High-risk groups include intravenous drug users, sexually promiscuous people, homosexuals, health-care professionals who come into contact with blood and body fluids, prisoners and other people who are institutionalized, and babies born to mothers with the disease. Infected babies generally have a more chronic form of the disease. Babies born to Alaskan natives, Pacific Islanders and first-generation immigrant mothers from Asia, the Middle East, Africa and Eastern Europe show the highest incidence rates. Pregnant women can be tested for hepatitis B and, if positive, their infants can be given hepatitis immune globulin (HGIB) at birth.

Vaccine History & Effectiveness: Hepatitis B is a new-generation, genetically-engineered recombinant DNA vaccine. In 1991, it became the first and only vaccine recommended for newborns (the first dose is given within the first 12 hours of life). This is curious because newborns are *not* at high risk for the disease. However, public health officials and doctors were unsuccessful at persuading adults in high-risk groups to get the vaccine. Thus, the motivation for such early vaccination appears to be that newborns are accessible (meaning that they are on medical turf and therefore present "an opportunity to vaccinate").

Vaccine Risks: The vaccine has been associated with severe, debilitating and life-threatening reactions. In France, the vaccine has been discontinued due to evidence that it can cause neurological disorders. Dr. Tenpenny has criticized the hepatitis B vaccine as being the most neurotoxic vaccine on the market, with more than 45 different types of reactions reported. The NVIC released figures in early 2001 showing that the number of hepatitis B vaccine-associated adverse events and deaths reported in U.S. children under the age of 14 is exceptionally high (827 in 1996), significantly outnumbering the reported cases of hepatitis B disease in that same age group (279).

Human Papillomavirus (HPV)

Agent: a virus transmitted through sexual contact; most common sexually transmitted disease in the U.S. About 98 percent of HPV infections resolve on their own within two years.

Disease Symptoms: genital warts and cancer (including cervical, vulvar, vaginal, anal and throat cancer).

Vaccine History & Effectiveness: The HPV vaccines Gardasil (approved in 2006), Cervarix (approved in 2009) and Gardasil 9 (approved in 2014) are genetically-engineered vaccines designed to prevent cervical and other sexually-transmitted types of cancer. Gardasil targets the four most common strains of HPV known to be associated with cervical cancer (more than 100 strains have been identified). Cervarix targets fewer cervical-cancer-causing strains, but seems to offer better protection from genital warts than Gardasil. And now Gardasil 9 targets nine strains of HPV. HPV vaccines are given as a series of three shots over six months and recommended for preteen girls and boys at 11 or 12 years of age.

Vaccine Risks: After Gardasil was licensed, there were thousands of reports of sudden collapse and unconsciousness within 24 hours. Seizures, muscle pain and weakness, disabling fatigue, Guillain Barre Syndrome, facial paralysis, brain inflammation, rheumatoid arthritis, lupus, blood clots, optic neuritis, multiple sclerosis, strokes, heart and other serious health problems, including death, have been reported. By the end of 2013, there were a total of 29,918 reaction reports made to VAERS associated with Gardasil vaccinations, including 140 deaths, and a total of 2,652 adverse reaction reports associated with Cervarix vaccinations, including 13 deaths.

Let's put the HPV cervical cancer risk in perspective. The death rate from cervical cancer in the U.S. is 3 out of 100,000 women. The rate of serious adverse events from Gardasil is about 3.4 per 100,000 doses. According to Dr. Christiane Northrup,

> *"Since their approval in 2006, nothing has convinced me that the benefits of the HPV vaccines outweigh the risks, which are significant. And now I'm troubled by another aspect. Did you know that women require a booster shot every five years for Gardasil and every seven years for Cervarix? Or that no one seems to know whether the HPV vaccines provide coverage to males for more than two years? Yet, the pharmaceutical companies along with the mainstream medical community, tout these vaccines as if they provide long-term protection."* [http://www.drnorthrup.com/the-hpv-vaccine-what-you-need-to-know-today/#sthash.Dfr8fnKz.dpuf]

Northrup goes on to suggest three steps which she believes offer safer protection against cervical cancer:

1. Boost your immunity and adopt lifestyle habits that support your health overall. This includes making sure your vitamin D levels are optimal. Studies show that those with optimal vitamin D levels cut their cancer risk, from all causes, in half.
2. Get regular pap smears, every three to five years.
3. Practice safe sex.

Furthermore, she suggests that if you're already infected, don't get an HPV vaccine. In 98 percent of cases, the body's own immune system will clear the virus from the system within two years. And finally, if you still plan to vaccinate, question the guidelines.

> *"Since Merck received FDA approval in 2006, they have marketed Gardasil to nine-year-old girls. Recently, they began marketing to eleven-year-old boys. It makes no sense to give your child a proven harmful substance to protect her from something she likely won't even come in contact with for several years. Most HPV is contracted in young adults between the ages of 16 and 26, which is the optimal time for vaccination if, at that time, you believe the benefits outweigh the risks"* [same source as above].

Influenza

Agent: virus transmitted like the common cold; there are different strains of influenza around the world, with a different strain predominating each year.

Disease Symptoms: fever, headache, body aches, sore throat, vomiting, diarrhea, stuffy nose, runny nose and cough; complications can include dehydration and pneumonia.

Vaccine History & Effectiveness: An inactivated injectable vaccine and a live-viral nasal spray are available. The nasal vaccine is more effective, but carries a greater risk of side effects. Each year, different viral influenza strains are used to cover the predicted strains for the coming year. The strains chosen each year are based on scientists' best guess and are not always accurately predicted.

Dr. Sears notes that the most common source of influenza death statistics is the MMWR database which combines deaths from influenza and pneumonia into one group, grossly over-estimating the overall number of deaths each year from influenza and giving the false impression that thousands of infants die from influenza each year. These are the statistics read by most doctors and repeated in the mainstream media. However, the reality is that 90 percent of the mortality in this country is in the 65-and-older age group.

Vaccine Risks: About two-thirds of recipients report one or more typical influenza symptoms within a week of vaccination. Allergic reactions have occurred. People who are allergic to eggs or who have had Guillain-Barre syndrome should not get the influenza shot according to the package inserts. Other neurological reactions include encephalopathy, facial and arm paralysis, and visual problems. The following people should not get the live-virus nasal spray vaccine: children under age 17 who have a medical condition requiring them to routinely take aspirin (can mix with the virus and cause a life-threatening reaction called known as Reye's Syndrome) and people with chronic lung, heart or immune system disease (the killed injected virus is thought to be safer for this group). For about three weeks after the nasal spray is given, the recipient is considered slightly contagious to close contacts. Finally, the influenza vaccine contains more chemicals than most vaccines (see Sears' book for details) and even the pro-vaccine Dr. Sears summarizes his judgment that "influenza isn't a disease to live in fear of."

Measles (MMR)

Agent: a viral infection of the respiratory system, eyes and skin.

Disease Symptoms: high fever, cough, runny nose, sore and sensitive eyes, Koplik's spots (tiny bluish-white spots, surrounded by redness on inside of the cheeks), swollen lymph nodes and characteristic rash of face, spreading over the trunk and body. The disease confers permanent immunity; the infected person will not contract it again. Complications include: ear infections, pneumonia, subacute sclerosing panencephalitis which causes intellectual deterioration, convulsive seizures, motor abnormalities and death. Previously healthy children usually recover without incident, but measles can be dangerous in malnourished populations living in underdeveloped countries, especially populations newly exposed to the virus; also dangerous in impoverished communities in developed countries where there is inadequate nutrition, sanitation and health care. Complications are more likely in infants, adults and anyone with a compromised immune system.

Treatment: The disease will run its course. Cool sponge baths, lotions to relieve itchy rash and hydration during the fever are recommended support therapies. Vitamin A supplementation with cod liver oil has been shown to reduce incidence of complications, while *use of fever-suppressing drugs is linked with an increased risk of complications* (Miller, *Vaccines: Are They Really Safe and Effective*).

Vaccine History & Effectiveness: The vaccine was created in 1963. It is a live-viral vaccine (along with mumps, rubella and chickenpox vaccines). Unlike bacteria, live-viruses cannot grow in mediums, but only in living cells. Oral polio, for example, is grown in kidney tissues of the African green monkey and the MMR in chick embryos. Tissue from aborted human fetuses has been used to grow the rubella virus.

From 1915 to 1958—before the measles vaccine was introduced—the death rate from measles in the U.S. had already declined on its own by 98 percent. The post-vaccine era death rate is almost identical to the pre-vaccine death rate. According to the World Health Organization, vaccinated people are actually more likely to contract measles than non-vaccinated people. Consider the following: in 1984, 58 percent of all school-aged children in the U.S. who contracted measles were adequately vaccinated and in 1988, that same figure jumped to 69 percent and in 1989, it jumped to 89 percent; in 1985, in Corpus Christi, TX, a measles outbreak occurred among a population that was 99 percent vaccinated; in 1986, there was an outbreak in Dane County, WI where 96 percent of the cases were in vaccinated people; in 1995, 56 percent of all reported measles cases in the U.S. were in previously vaccinated people. (Miller, *Vaccines: Are They Really Safe and Effective?*).

Use of the measles vaccine has caused a demographic shift in the pattern of infection. Instead of contracting the disease in childhood, most cases are now found among adolescents and young adults. Complications of measles at this age can be much more serious and long-lasting. At the other end of the spectrum, many more infants are now infected than ever before. This trend is expected to continue unabated due to the growing number of new mothers who were themselves vaccinated and therefore unable to pass on any immunity to their infants (the limited vaccine-conferred immunity being much weaker than true immunity gained from having had measles). When mothers have true immunity from the disease, antibodies are passed to the baby at birth and are protective through 15 months of age. Prior to introduction of the vaccine, it was extremely rare for an infant to have measles, but by 1992, at least 28 percent of all reported measles cases were in infants. Similarly, by 1977, 60 percent of all cases were in persons over the age of 10 and 26 percent were in persons 15 years and older (compared to a pre-vaccine era rate of 10 percent in this population) (Miller, *Vaccines: Are They Really Safe and Effective?*).

Vaccine Risks: Adverse reactions include an extensive list of ailments affecting nearly every body system—blood, lymphatic, digestive, cardiovascular, immune, nervous, respiratory and sensory; learning difficulties, mental retardation, aseptic meningitis, seizure disorders, paralysis and death have been linked to the vaccine; suspected links with the development of eczema and chronic arthritis for the MMR vaccine taken as a whole.

The MMR vaccine has also been strongly linked as a possible etiology for *autistic regression* in previously developmentally normal children. This link has been dismissed by vaccine proponents based on research that is rife with conflict of interest (i.e., the vaccine manufacturer designs "research" that "debunks" multiple parental reports of sudden regression after administration of the vaccine—the conclusions are foregone). Autistic regression is characterized by a pattern of loss of speech, language and social skills, accompanied by bizarre behaviors. Additional symptoms include excessive thirst, bowel disturbances (autistic enterocolitis), self-injury and a self-limited diet associated with cravings for particular foods. Asthma, eczema, hay fever and recurrent upper respiratory infections are prominent features of the autistic regression symptom picture as well.

Autistic regression is different from the classic, early onset form of autism which typically manifests in the first and second year of life as the child does not develop in the way of normal siblings and peers. Because diagnosis of early onset autism often coincides in time with administration of the MMR vaccine, claims that the MMR *causes* autism have been dismissed as "coincidence." One only need to read the magnitude of testimonials by parents who describe a previously normal child descending into the hell of autism shortly after receiving the MMR vaccine to question whether due diligence has been done to assure that there truly and absolutely is *no connection* between autism and the MMR. In my judgment, the jury is still out on this issue. For more information, read this recent article by investigative journalist Sheryl Attkinson, "What the News Isn't Saying about Vaccine-Autism Studies [http://sharylattkisson.com/what-the-news-isnt-saying-about-vaccine-autism-studies].

From an epidemiological perspective, increases in the number of autism cases are temporally consistent with the introduction of the vaccine. This holds true in other countries as well and takes into consideration changes in diagnostic criteria for autism (an excuse often given for the rising number of autism cases by vaccine proponents).

Dr. Sears recommends that the MMR vaccine should only be given when the child's digestive system is at peak health. If the child has taken antibiotics in the past few weeks or is experiencing diarrhea, then the vaccine should be delayed till a later time while probiotic supplementation is given and digestive health is restored (see pages 81–2 for more information). Furthermore, *this vaccine should not be administered to women who are about to become pregnant, are pregnant or breastfeeding.*

Meningococcal Disease

Agent: bacterium causes an infection that runs through the bloodstream infecting various body organs and can spread to the brain causing meningitis; transmitted like the common cold.

Disease symptoms: Rapid onset of aches and fever, can progress to full-blown meningitis within 24 hours (high fever, severe headache, neck stiffness, vomiting and red pinpoint dots that progress to become larger purple splotches all over the body). Highest incidence in infants six months to two years of age, college students living in dormitories and military personnel living in barracks. Overall mortality rate is 10 percent; 20 percent among affected college students. Permanent disability among survivors occurs about 15 percent of the time and includes nerve damage, hearing loss and rare loss of a limb due to infection.

Vaccine History & Effectiveness: One of the newer vaccines, the meningococcal vaccine was licensed in 2005 and has been found to be about 58 percent effective within two to five years after administration. In 2011, the CDC recommended that all 16-year-olds get a booster dose.

Vaccine Risks: Adverse reactions include irritability, abnormal crying, fever, drowsiness, fatigue, injection site pain and swelling, sudden loss of consciousness, diarrhea, headache, joint pain, Guillain Barre Syndrome, brain inflammation, convulsions and facial palsy. By August 2012, VAERS had recorded more than 2,300 serious health problems, injuries and hospitalizations following meningococcal shots, including 39 deaths with about 40 percent of the deaths occurring in children under age six.

Mumps (MMR)

Agent: a mild viral infection of the salivary glands beneath the ears, along the jaw.

Disease Symptoms: swollen and painful glands, fever, headache, muscle aches, fatigue, vomiting; testicles, ovaries and breasts may become inflamed; an estimated 30 percent of cases go unnoticed; disease confers permanent immunity, the infected person will not contract it again. Rarely are there any complications in childhood cases. The disease is more severe in teenagers and adults. Approximately 20 percent of post-pubescent males experience orchitis (inflammation of the testes), though sterility following orchitis is very rare as usually only one testicle is involved. Other, extremely rare complications include transient meningitis and temporary hearing loss.

Treatment: Allow the disease to run its course; medical intervention is rarely required.

Vaccine History & Effectiveness: The vaccine was introduced in the late 1960s. Today, it is one component of the MMR vaccine and it is a live viral vaccine. Artificial immunity conferred by the vaccine is notoriously unreliable. Those who escape the disease in childhood, through successful inoculation, but develop the mumps later in life, face a more intense version of the disease. Since widespread use of the vaccine, the disease has shifted into the older higher-risk group, similar to what resulted from the measles vaccine. For example, prior to introduction of the vaccine, only 8 percent of cases occurred in individuals 15 years or older; by 1987, this number jumped to 38 percent of cases. Furthermore, when outbreaks have occurred, vaccinated persons have been more than twice as likely as unvaccinated persons to contract the disease (Miller, *Vaccines: Are They Really Safe and Effective?*).

Vaccine Risks: Adverse reactions include fever, seizures, nerve deafness, meningitis (1 in 1,000 doses), encephalitis and diabetes. Suspected links with the development of eczema and chronic arthritis for the MMR vaccine taken as a whole.

Dr. Sears recommends that the MMR vaccine should only be given when the child's digestive system is at peak health. If the child has taken antibiotics in the past few weeks, or is experiencing diarrhea, then the vaccine should be delayed till a later time.

Consider: Visionary pediatrician Dr. Robert Mendelsohn commented that if mumps vaccine is given to protect adult males from orchitis and possible sterility, and not to prevent mumps in children, then why not just give it to males who have not developed natural immunity by puberty? And what is the *medical rationale* for vaccinating girls against mumps?

Pertussis (Whooping Cough) (DTaP)

Agent: bacterial respiratory infection.

Disease Symptoms: fever, difficulty breathing, characteristic cough resulting from victim trying to catch their breath during episodes, vomiting after attacks; convulsions from lack of oxygen in severe cases; recovery takes two to three months.

Treatment: Antibiotics can be used to kill the bacteria so that the person is no longer contagious; this can stop spread of the disease. However, damage to the airway produces weeks of coughing even after the bacteria are gone.

Vaccine History & Effectiveness: The vaccine was made in 1936 and in general use by the mid-1940s. Pertussis was the second component of the DPT vaccine. It was made from killed whole-cell pertussis bacteria which is so highly toxic in its pure form that scientists have used it to induce experimental brain-damage in laboratory animals. In 1991, the acellular pertussis (aP) vaccine was approved for use by the FDA. It is considered to be a safer vaccine, with many of the impurities and toxins of the whole-cell version removed. In 1996, the aP replaced the whole cell vaccine. It is not possible to get the aP as a single vaccine; it is currently only manufactured as a component of the DTaP vaccine.

It is interesting to note that, from 1900 to 1935, before pertussis vaccine was available, the death rate from pertussis fell 79 percent in the United States. A 1989 study reported in the *Journal of Pediatrics* revealed that the effectiveness of the pertussis vaccine may be as low as 40 percent. In 1989, the NVIC reported that during a ten-month period in 1984, 49 percent of all whooping cough victims between three months and six years of age had been previously vaccinated. So the overall effectiveness of the pertussis vaccine has been called into question.

Vaccine Risks: The whole-cell pertussis vaccine was one of the most reactive vaccines ever created and was known to cause high fever, severe pain and swelling at the injection site, diarrhea, projectile vomiting, sleepiness, persistent high-pitched screaming, seizures, convulsions, shock, breathing problems, brain damage and death. In 1998, 57 deaths were reported to VAERS as having been caused by the pertussis vaccine. Unfortunately, similar severe reactions to aP have also been reported, though not as many.

Pneumococcal Disease (Pc)

Agent: bacterium that causes a wide range of illnesses; transmitted by inhaling the respiratory droplets of an infected person.

Disease Symptoms: mild cold symptoms and ear infections; complications include pneumonia, bloodstream infections and meningitis with a 20–30 percent fatality rate, higher in elderly populations

Vaccine History & Effectiveness: The vaccine was introduced in 2001. The CDC estimated that prior to introduction of the vaccine, there were about 60,000 reported cases each year; about 17,000 cases were in children younger than five years of age. While these numbers have decreased by about half since introduction of the vaccine, an increase in strains of the Pc germ not covered by the vaccine (up to 96 percent of cases in one hospital) has been noted. Dr. Sears estimates that there about 10,000 severe cases of Pc disease in young children each year in the U.S. and another 20,000–30,000 cases in adults. Approximately 2,000–3,000 cases per year are of the severe, antibiotic-resistant variety and occur mostly in infants under age two and the elderly.

Treatment: severe infections require hospitalization with IV antibiotics; minor infections with oral antibiotics.

Vaccine Risks: standard reactions include fever, crying, vomiting, diarrhea, poor appetite, sleepiness, headache, body aches and rash; isolated seizures have been noted.

Polio

Agent: intestinal virus that attacks the brain and spinal cord.

Disease Symptoms: fever, headache, sore throat, vomiting; complications include stiffness of neck and back, muscle weakness, painful joints, paralysis of limbs or paralysis of respiratory muscles, which can be fatal. The wild polio virus produces no symptoms in more than 90 percent of those exposed to it. Paralytic polio occurs in about 1 percent of those infected. Risks for developing the paralytic form of polio, after exposure, include:

- fatigue and strenuous exercise
- injections or other trauma to the limbs
- a family history of paralytic polio
- tonsillectomy (greatly increases the risk; it is interesting to note that tonsillectomy was the most commonly performed elective surgical procedure of the 1950s, which was coincident with the U.S. polio epidemic)

Treatment: For the person who suffers from paralysis of the lungs, hospitalization in intensive care is required until the paralysis wears off.

Vaccine History & Effectiveness: In 1955, Dr. Jonas Salk developed the killed-virus or inactivated polio vaccine (IPV). It produces blood antibodies, but limited intestinal immunity. In 1959, Dr. Albert Sabin developed the live-virus oral polio vaccine (OPV) which produces a high level of both blood and intestinal antibodies.

From 1923 to 1953 (before the Salk vaccine was introduced) the polio death rate in the United States had declined by 47 percent and was dropping fast all over the world. When the live-virus vaccine was introduced, the standards for defining polio were changed. By the old tally, only 24 hours of paralysis were needed to qualify as a polio infection. The new standard required 60 days of paralysis to be included as a confirmed polio case. In addition, a similar illness, aseptic meningitis—previously included in the old polio standard—was dropped from the new standard. This procedure radically skewed the statistics, creating the impression of a drastic reduction in polio after the introduction of the live-viral vaccine.

There have been no documented cases of wild polio in the U.S. since 1979 and none in the entire Western Hemisphere since 1994. In 1976, Dr. Salk testified that the live-virus vaccine had been the principle, if not the sole, cause of all reported polio cases in the U.S. since 1961. According to the CDC, every case of polio contracted in the U.S. from 1980 to 1989 was caused by the vaccine. Use of the OPV was subsequently discontinued in the U.S. in 2000.

Vaccine Risks: The IPV is associated with arthritis, central nervous system damage and chronic fatigue syndrome.

Rotavirus

Agent: intestinal virus that causes vomiting and diarrhea; transmitted through contact with the stools or saliva of an infected person; increased risk in daycare settings.

Disease Symptoms: fever, vomiting, diarrhea lasting more than a few days, up to weeks; primary complication is dehydration; death from dehydration is a greater risk in third world countries where emergency IV therapy may not be readily available.

Treatment: There are no medications to fight rotavirus, though IV therapy is an effective support to prevent dehydration. Probiotic powder can shorten the course of the disease and it is recommended that infants be taken off of cow's milk or formulas based on cow's milk while ill and substitute soy-based formulas instead. Breast milk, of course, is the ideal hydration for babies.

Vaccine History & Effectiveness: The rotavirus vaccine was introduced in 1998. Just four months after the CDC issued recommendations that all babies be injected with three doses of the newly licensed vaccine to prevent infant diarrhea, the CDC suspended use of the vaccine. It seems that a number of infants required surgery to correct a condition called intussusception (a type of bowel obstruction in which the bowel telescopes in on itself) within one week of receiving the vaccine. The number of reported cases grew from 15 to 104, including two deaths, before the manufacturer withdrew the vaccine from the market. And all of this for an illness that is highly treatable with readily-available rehydration therapy in the U.S. and which does not cause widespread death among U.S. children. Retrospective analysis of VRBPAC records show that committee members responsible for voting on licensure were aware that intussusception was a risk factor from the clinical trial data, but determined that the risk was not statistically significant.

A new rotavirus vaccine is now on the market and intussusception is still listed as a side effect. Dr. Sears dismisses this risk in his book, claiming coincidence. At the same time, he lists the symptoms of intussusception, which is a medical emergency:

> *"extreme fussiness, vomiting, bloody stools and episodes of intense abdominal pain ... infants draw the knees up to the abdomen for several minutes while in pain, then relax into lethargy ... continues in waves that can last as long as thirty minutes at a time."*

Vaccine Risks: standard side effects, seizures, intussusception and live viral shedding in the stools for up to 15 days post vaccination has been noted.

Rubella (German Measles) (MMR)

Agent: a mild viral infection of the respiratory system, skin and lymph nodes.

Disease Symptoms: runny nose, low fever, sore throat, swelling of lymph nodes of head and neck; characteristic rash on face, limbs and trunk; swelling and pain in the joints; disease often goes undetected and passes as a cold; most cases confer permanent immunity; rare incidence of recurrence in the same person.

Complications: Rubella is a very mild childhood disease which requires no treatment, but is known to pose danger to a fetus if the mother contracts it during the first trimester of pregnancy. In these cases, it is associated with an increased incidence of miscarriage, birth defects and mental retardation.

Vaccine History & Effectiveness: The vaccine was developed in 1969. It is a live viral vaccine and is administered as a component of the MMR vaccine. It has proven unreliable, lending immunity to a young girl for a time after vaccination, but increasing her chances of contracting the disease at a later time in life, possibly during pregnancy when the risk is highest. Dr. Mendelsohn cites a study of young vaccinated girls, 36 percent of whom had no evidence of immunity by adolescence. Another study, reported in a 1973 issue of the *Australian Journal of Medical Technology,* reveals that 80 percent of army recruits contracted rubella within four months after receiving the vaccine. Prior to introduction of the vaccine, 85 percent of adults were naturally immune to rubella. After widespread acceptance of the vaccine, 15 percent of the adult population remains susceptible to rubella.

The epidemiological shifts in the disease are similar to what has happened with measles and mumps. Prior to introduction of the vaccine, 23 percent of all cases occurred in persons 15 years or older; by 1990, 81 percent of all cases occurred in this age group, with the highest incidence occurring in persons 15 to 29 years old, the primary childbearing years (Miller, *Vaccines: Are They Really Safe and Effective?*).

Finally, a review of the effectiveness of the rubella vaccine shows that, while the number of rubella cases overall has declined since introduction of the vaccine, the incidence of congenital rubella syndrome (CRS) has remained constant. Furthermore, when the number of fetuses aborted due to CRS is taken into consideration, the actual incidence of CRS has increased, possibly as much as 10 percent or more (Miller, *Vaccines: Are They Really Safe and Effective?*).

Vaccine Risks: The vaccine is associated with arthritis, central nervous system damage, chronic fatigue syndrome, diabetes, anaphylaxis and death. There are suspected links with the development of eczema and chronic arthritis for the MMR vaccine taken as a whole. In a 1986 study of adult women who received the vaccine, 55 percent developed arthritis or joint pain within four weeks of vaccination (Miller, *Vaccines: Are They Really Safe and Effective?*). Sears states that:

> *"Women who already suffer from arthritis or have a strong family history of rheumatoid arthritis should be aware of the potential for arthritis when they get this shot and weigh the risk of being susceptible to rubella during future pregnancies versus the risk of arthritis side effects from the shot."*

As mentioned above, Dr. Sears recommends that the MMR vaccine should only be given when the child's digestive system is at peak health. If the child has taken antibiotics in the past few weeks, or is experiencing diarrhea, then the vaccine should be delayed till a later time.

Consider: Mass vaccination campaigns to protect against rubella were never intended to protect vaccine recipients, but rather the fetuses of rubella-susceptible pregnant women. If a decision is made to not vaccinate against rubella, pre-adolescent girls can be tested for the presence of rubella antibodies through a simple blood test. If antibody tests do not indicate immunity to the disease, the vaccination decision can be reconsidered at this time.

Tetanus (DTaP)

Agent: an infection of the nervous system caused by a toxin produced by the tetanus bacterium which enters the bloodstream through a wound.

Disease Symptoms: toxin attacks spinal cord nerve cells that control muscle activity, resulting in rigid muscles and painful spasms, especially of the jaw (lockjaw); untreated cases can progress to convulsions and death. It is caused when the bacteria enters a wound that provides anaerobic (lacking oxygen) conditions, such as a deep puncture wound. The most common source of infection is soil contaminated with animal feces, especially horses.

Tetanus is extremely rare. The risk of tetanus goes up if a child lives on a farm, plays around horses or travels to a third-world country where hygiene is poor.

Urban children and infants and children under the age of two are at low risk of getting tetanus.

The following injuries are considered <u>high risk for tetanus</u>:

- wound is exposed to a high level of contamination such as barnyards or sewers
- wound is over 24 hours old at the time of first treatment
- wound contains unrecoverable debris or dead tissue

The following injuries are considered to pose a <u>moderate risk for tetanus</u>:

- wound is exposed to a moderate level of contamination such as wood, pavement or industrial areas
- any crush or puncture wound
- wound extends into the muscle
- human bites

<u>Vaccine History & Effectiveness</u>: The vaccine was introduced during World War II. It is a component of the DTaP vaccine and is made from the toxoid, much like the diphtheria vaccine. Tetanus cases in the U.S. military declined 99.8 percent from the Civil War to the end of World War II and were already in steep decline all over the civilized world by the time the vaccine was introduced. Nevertheless, the tetanus vaccine is considered to be one of the most effective vaccines on the market.

<u>Vaccine Risks</u>: Adverse reactions include: nerve damage to the inner ear, nervous system degeneration,

allergic shock reaction and loss of consciousness. *The risk of adverse vaccine reactions goes up if a person is over-immunized.* Three previous doses of the toxoid, with boosters given every ten years is the *maximum* recommended dose. There is a slight risk of hyper immunization when treated in a hospital emergency room, so parents are advised to keep accurate vaccine records and let older children know their status.

Note: *Tetanus vaccine is not effective if administered after an injury to someone who has not received a minimum of two previous doses of the vaccine.* In other words, one cannot forego the vaccine on the premise that they will get vaccinated if they suffer a high-risk injury. However, tetanus anti-toxin, also known as tetanus immune globulin, can be given to unvaccinated or under-vaccinated people (meaning those with less than two previous doses of the toxoid vaccine) who have suffered a high-risk or moderate-risk injury. The anti-toxin does not confer lasting immunity, but it does contain antibodies that will attack the tetanus bacteria. Combined with good wound hygiene, the anti-toxin provides good protection from tetanus (see also the section on Homeopathy).

Varicella Zoster (Chickenpox)

Agent: virus of the herpes family, clinically associated with herpes zoster (shingles), causing skin lesions.

Disease Symptoms: fever, loss of appetite, irritability; spots appearing all over the body form itchy blisters that go through a pustular stage before crusting over. It is a mild childhood disease with rare complications that include encephalitis and a severe strep infection of the lesions which is difficult to treat with antibiotics and may be life-threatening. Adults generally suffer more with the disease and complications are more common. In fact, the number of adults who require hospitalization due to chickenpox is 10–20 times greater than the number of children. As with other live-viral vaccines, widespread use of the herpes zoster vaccine is shifting the disease into the higher-risk groups.

Vaccine History & Effectiveness: The vaccine was finally licensed by the FDA in 1995. Developed decades earlier, a benefit-versus-risk analysis of the chickenpox vaccine had prevented it from being manufactured. In the nineties, however, policy makers decided that the vaccine should be mandated, not because the disease suddenly presented a greater threat to children, but because of the cost to society of parents' lost days from work, staying home to care for sick children. I remember seeing a full page promotional ad in the *New York Times* shortly after the chickenpox vaccine was licensed for use. Merck, the manufacturer, clearly understood that the first obstacle to widespread acceptance of this vaccine was public perception that chickenpox was not a disease to be feared. The ad featured a pair of concerned parents flanking the hospital bed of a young child receiving IV fluids. The accompanying caption read "We never knew chickenpox could be so serious."

Vaccine Risks: Adverse reactions include pain, soreness and swelling at the injection site; chickenpox lesions at the injection site and elsewhere on the body; high fever, upper respiratory infection and more.

ADVERSE REACTIONS TO VACCINATIONS

Vaccine Ingredients

For more information about how vaccines are made, see the Sears' book and publications by Neil Miller's Think Twice Global Vaccine Institute. Vaccines may have the following ingredients in varying combinations and quantities:

- live viruses
- bacteria
- egg protein
- antibiotics
- diseased animal matter
- cells/tissues from aborted fetuses
- toxic substances and known neurotoxins and carcinogens including aluminum, formaldehyde and trace amounts of mercury

Aluminum in Vaccines

The Sears' book is particularly helpful in its analysis of each vaccine brand for potentially harmful ingredients, with emphasis placed on minimizing exposure to aluminum. Aluminum is a known neurotoxin that has been linked with Alzheimer's disease. If choosing to vaccinate, parents may want to consider limiting aluminum exposure by allowing only one or two aluminum-containing vaccines to be given at a time. Certain brands contain more than others and combination vaccines may deliver an especially high amount. Check the Sears' book for details, including an alternate vaccination schedule designed to reduce exposure to aluminum. Another great resource is the NVIC website which has a Vaccine Ingredients Calculator whereby parents can calculate vaccine ingredients for potential toxic exposure and print out an individualized vaccination plan [http://www.vaccine-tlc.org].

Mercury in Vaccines

There is no debate from any quarter that mercury is bad for you. It is well known to be a neurotoxin. In vaccines, mercury is in the form of thimerosal, a highly toxic mercury compound widely used as a vaccine preservative. Since 2001, all vaccines routinely recommended for children younger than six years of age have been thimerosal-free, with the exception of the inactivated influenza vaccine. It is important to note that most vaccines still contain trace amounts of mercury, including the so-called "mercury-free" vaccines. Thimerosal is routinely used in the manufacture of vaccines and injectables but the FDA does not require it be listed as an ingredient if it is used during the manufacturing process, only if it is added afterwards.

Vaccine Risks

Vaccine reactions fall into the following broad categories:

- *Local reactions* include pain and swelling at the injection site.
- *Mild to moderate systemic reactions* include infection at the injection site, fever, decreased

appetite, vomiting, diarrhea, headaches, body aches, rash, drowsiness and fretfulness.

- *Severe systemic reactions* include convulsions, seizure disorders, collapse, high fever (105 or more), persistent uncontrollable crying for more than three hours, high-pitched screaming, brain disease, brain damage, paralysis, central nervous system damage and death. While admitting that adverse vaccine reactions are notoriously under-reported, Dr. Sears calculates the risk of a serious vaccine reaction (based on data that was reported in 1991 through 2001) as follows:

  - 1 in 100,000 chance for each separate vaccine
  - 1 in 35,000 chance for each round of vaccines
  - 1 in 2,600 chance for entire 12-year vaccine schedule

Since babies are now given approximately twice the number of injections as they were given in the decade for which Sears did his calculations, the risks are likely significantly higher than noted above.

- *Long-term damage* includes low resistance to infections; allergies, asthma and juvenile-onset diabetes; suspected links with the unexplained and alarming rise in cases of autism, learning disabilities and attention deficit disorders, as well as auto-immune disorders such as AIDS, chronic fatigue syndrome and cancer. The risk here is unknown at this time.

It is important to understand the indoctrination of thinking among U.S. doctors when it comes to vaccine reactions which can be summarized as follows: There is no distinct syndrome associated with vaccine administration and, therefore, many temporally associated adverse events probably represent background illness rather than illness caused by the vaccine. For example, the DTaP may stimulate or precipitate inevitable symptoms of underlying central nervous system disorders such as seizures, infantile spasms, epilepsy or SIDS. By chance alone, it is claimed, these cases will be deemed to be temporally related to administration of the vaccine. Thereby, the responsibility for the alleged adverse event is placed on the genetically defective child and written off.

Vaccines and Autism

Autism rates in the U.S. have grown from 1 in 2,000 before 1990 to 1 in 150 in 2002 to 1 in 68 in 2014. Despite media reports to the contrary, it is *not* true that vaccines have been proven to *not* be a factor in the autism epidemic. What *is* true is that powerful vested interests rallied to discredit the work of Dr. Andrew Wakefield (published in the British medical journal *The Lancet* in 1998) whose research suggested that there might be an association between vaccine-induced chronic inflammation in the body and developmental delays. See point #6 in the article *First They Came for the Anti-Vaxxers* by Bretigne Shaffer, briefly summarized on page 109 for more links to research suggesting a causal link between vaccines and autism. The jury is out on this one.

Vaccines and Ear Infections
The following vaccines/brands are known to *cause* ear infections according to information contained in the package inserts: Biavax, Engerix, Tetramune, Prevnar, Varivax and the MMR vaccine.

Preventing Vaccine Reactions

General Precautions
Ask yourself the following questions *before* vaccinating:

- Is my child sick right now? (If the answer is yes, *do resist* pressure to vaccinate.)
- Has my child had a previous bad reaction to a vaccine?
- Is there a personal or family history of vaccine reactions, convulsions, neurological disorders, severe allergies or immune system disorders?
- Do I know if my child is at high risk of reacting?
- Have I identified the least toxic brand of the vaccine? (Does my current pediatrician use the least toxic brand or will he/she order it for me?)
- Am I fully informed about vaccine side effects?
- Do I know how to identify a vaccine reaction?
- Do I know how to report a vaccine reaction?
- Do I have a record of the vaccine manufacturer's name and lot number?

Essential Pre-Vaccination Reading
- Vaccine Package Inserts. These manufacturer's warnings contain the most complete and updated material on vaccine effects and are essential pre-vaccine reading. *Legally, it is your responsibility*

to read package inserts because court precedent is such that if a child is damaged in a way that the insert adequately warns of, the manufacturer cannot be held liable. Pay special attention to warnings contained in sections titled "adverse reactions," "contra-indications" and "warnings." If your child falls into a high-risk-for-reacting category, these contraindications constitute the grounds for a medical exemption from mandatory vaccination. Package inserts are available here: http://www.immunize.org/packageinserts/.

- Vaccine Information Statements (VIS) by the CDC. The law requires your doctor to provide you with these brief warnings regarding vaccinations. These government-required statements are a shortened version of the complete contraindications and warnings for the vaccines. They can be found here: http://www.cdc.gov/vaccines/hcp/vis/. At the very least, read the VIS, if not the package inserts.

Repeating Vaccines after a Serious Reaction
Vaccine guidelines, as well as most doctors, recommend that a vaccine should be continued, even after a serious reaction has occurred, because the benefits outweigh the risks. Really? *Vaccine literature demonstrates that severe reactions tend to become even worse with subsequent shots* and the vaccine package inserts themselves recommend *against* repeating a vaccine after an allergic reaction has occurred. At the very least, cautious consumers should consider giving a previously-reactive vaccine by itself, without other simultaneous

vaccines. In addition, reactivity tends to run in families, so parents are advised to be cautious about proceeding with vaccinating siblings of a highly-reactive child.

Vitamin C Supplementation
Because vaccination has been demonstrated to wipe out vitamin C stores in the body, many authors recommend vitamin C supplementation before and after vaccination. I have seen recommendations for dosages of up to 3,000 mg daily for one week before and one week after vaccination. See the article on *Stimulating a Weakened Immune System* by Jane Sheppard (on page 80) for age-adjusted dosages. While overdosing with vitamin C is not toxic, it can cause loose bowel movements. Dr. Sears' specific recommendations are less aggressive: once per day for five days starting on the day of the shots; infants should get 150 milligrams, toddlers and preschoolers 250 milligrams, and older kids and teens 500 milligrams.

Vitamin A Supplementation
Vitamin A supports neurologic health as well as regulating the immune system's response to infections. Dr. Sears cites researchers who believe that vitamin A can play a role in protecting the brain from vaccine side effects. He recommends one dose a day for three days prior to vaccination and continuing for ten days after. Infant dose is 1500 IUs daily, 2500 IUs for toddlers and preschoolers, and 5000 IUs for older kids and teens. Best food source of vitamin A is cod liver oil. Unlike vitamin C, parents should take care not to exceed recommended dosages of vitamin A. In addition, cod liver oil should not be given to babies under the age of

nine months due to an increased risk of triggering a fish allergy.

Probiotic Supplementation

Probiotics are healthful bacteria that normally live in the intestines. These bacteria help to balance naturally occurring yeast in the system as well as playing a critical role in regulating the immune system. When antibiotics are used, they do not discriminate between healthful and harmful bacteria in the system. Thus, after a course of antibiotics, the body is unbalanced, often favoring yeast overgrowth and weakened intestinal health (a bad time to vaccinate). The beneficial bacteria can be re-colonized through probiotic supplementation to optimize health. In addition, Dr. Sears recommends probiotic supplementation for a week before and several weeks after vaccinating. See pages 81–2 for more information.

Never Vaccinate a Sick Child

Be aware that the public health agenda tends to override other concerns and therefore may not be in the best interest of *your* child. Each doctor's office visit or ER interaction provides "an opportunity to vaccinate" for the pro-vaccine care provider. The rationale is that some children are unvaccinated through parental neglect rather than conscious and informed decision making. Each interface with the medical system then, presents an opportunity to extend vaccination coverage rates. The fact that the child is in the doctor's office or ER because they are sick or in trauma, is not considered a sufficient deterrent to delay vaccination where the assumed benefits outweigh the risks. Vaccine package inserts that warn against giving a vaccine when fever is present notwithstanding, politics override common sense. Thus, parents should be prepared to be pressured on this topic whenever interfacing with the medical system. Your only protection is to *know your rights!* You do not have to cave to pressure to vaccinate when your child is at greater risk of reacting to vaccines or at any other time.

If choosing to vaccinate, it makes sense to do so when your child is at peak health. See chapter on *Enhancing the Immune System Naturally* for more information on optimizing your child's immune system—good advice whether you choose to vaccinate or not.

Legal Recourse for Adverse Vaccine Reactions

The National Childhood Vaccine Injury Act (NCVIA) of 1986

As a result of this legislation, persons injured by vaccines and families of persons killed by vaccines are prohibited from suing vaccine manufacturers for vaccine-associated deaths or injuries until they file a claim with the National Vaccine Injury Compensation Program (NVICP). In other words, the federal government has assumed liability for vaccine damage. According to Kristine Severyn of the Vaccine Policy Institute (an Ohio organization that is no longer active),

> *"The program has three major drawbacks. First, it shifts vaccine liability from manufacturers, where it belongs, to the taxpayer. Second, it destroys incentives for vaccine manufacturers to improve existing products. After all, once a vaccine is licensed and mandated for everyone*

*and the government covers liability costs, there
is little incentive for a manufacturer to make it
safer. This leads to the third drawback, namely,
providing major profit incentives for drug
companies to market new vaccines."*

Vaccine Adverse Events Reporting System (VAERS)

The NCVIA also created VAERS to track adverse
events around the country [https://vaers.hhs.gov/index].
VAERS receives 12,000–17,000 reports each year. Of
these reports, an estimated 15 percent are serious
adverse reactions. Annually, 120 deaths are reported.
And, while these numbers are concerning, *it is well
known that adverse events are significantly under-
reported.* An estimated one in ten reactions are reported
to the VAERS.

National Vaccine Injury Compensation Program (NVICP)

Unfortunately this system, originally designed to protect
consumers, has become adversarial. Since 1989, 4,022
compensation awards have been made while 9,882
(approximately 70 percent) have been dismissed. Parents
can expect years of waiting and legal maneuvering.
Damage awards are paid by excise taxes on each dose of
vaccine.

Why are so many VICP claims dismissed?
According to Kristine Severyn,

> *"The VICP utilizes a narrow definition of
> vaccine injuries to award compensation known
> as the Vaccine Injury Table (VIT). If a vaccine
> injury is not listed on the VIT, the petitioner must
> prove that the vaccine directly caused the injury,*

a so-called 'causation in fact.' Such claims are nearly impossible to prove in the VICP."

In addition, all new vaccines added to the VICP in recent years have no conditions listed on the VIT, making it more difficult for petitioners to win VICP claims. Another limitation is that Congress has specified that in order for an injury to be compensable, it must be severe enough to last longer than six months.

Should you ever need to file a claim, I strongly recommend contacting the NVIC, a consumer group established by Barbara Loe Fisher, for help (see Resources). The NVIC publishes a booklet entitled *National Childhood Vaccine Injury Act of 1986. Public Law 99-660: The Compensation System and How It Works.* Read this booklet first if you need to file a claim. The Center also provides information and forms for filing a claim and can recommend legal counsel. For more information on the NVICP, see http://www.hrsa.gov/vaccinecompensation.

The Vaccine Injury Alliance (VIA)
The VIA is a consortium of law firms and legal professionals committed to helping families obtain compensation for vaccine-related injuries. The VIA is bringing its expertise, in both NVICP and traditional civil courts, to hundreds of adults and children from all over the country. For more information, go to http://www.vaccineinjury.org.

Vaccines & Informed Choice

ENHANCING THE IMMUNE SYSTEM NATURALLY

Do Germs Cause Disease?

History demonstrates that the specter of infectious disease, beyond the common childhood illnesses, can arise anywhere and at any time. Epidemics from exotic influenza strains to bubonic plague have left large populations dead or debilitated and may do so again without warning. But exposure is only half of the picture—one also needs to be susceptible to an infectious disease to contract it and there are always those whose constitution renders them immune to these periodic scourges.

Louis Pasteur, the father of the Germ Theory of Disease, confessed towards the end of his life that germs (bacteria, viruses) may not be the *cause* of disease after all, but rather a disease *symptom.* His contemporary, Antoine Bechamp, had believed that germs led to illness when the immune system was suppressed. Bechamp stated that the cause of disease was not simply the invading virus or bacteria, but *factors that compromise host resistance.* Immunity, in this view, equals the host's ability to maintain balance with the environment.

Nevertheless, Pasteur's Germ Theory continues to dominate the mainstream approach to disease and disease prevention. In this view, the infecting germ is the most important part of the equation. The germ becomes synonymous with the disease and, therefore, in order to maintain health, we must kill the germ or avoid contamination. Under Bechamp's theory, health is a matter of improving the internal environment—the "soil"—by addressing such factors as diet, lifestyle, toxicity, emotional state and mental stress. If the "soil" is improved, then the nature of the germs that are present is altered, as well as the toxins that the germs produce.

I found it interesting to note that, after a brief and scornful dismissal of those who might dare to question the Germ Theory, Dr. Sears wrote the following in *The Vaccine Book:*

> *"Do vaccines really cause side effects? Each vaccine has a list of reported side effects. But it's important to realize that we don't know whether these reactions are caused by a vaccine or just happen to occur randomly within a month of a vaccine. Reactions don't have to be proven to have been caused by a vaccine before they are added to the list of side effects. There's an old saying in science: temporality doesn't imply causality."*

It's a shame Dr. Sears can't apply this same principle to his thinking regarding the Germ Theory.

Nevertheless, the idea of individual susceptibility or predisposition to disease is acknowledged by every holistic healing modality, wherein treatment involves removing factors that inhibit the immune system from functioning properly, as well as stimulating the body to heal itself. So, if parents choose to reject vaccine technology as the sole means of protection against disease, what else can be done?

Understanding Disease Symptoms

In the orthodox view, symptoms are seen as "the problem" and treatment is aimed at making the symptoms go away. However, from a holistic perspective, the symptoms are the outward signs of a struggle that the immune system is waging. They are not the problem; they are the body's response to an underlying problem. For example, in a case of food poisoning, vomiting and diarrhea are the symptoms. They represent the body's effort to rid itself of the invading toxin, thereby minimizing the amount of the toxin that gets absorbed into the bloodstream. Medications that suppress vomiting and diarrhea may be given, but these have the effect of preventing the body from responding efficiently to the real problem.

In the case of an inflammatory response, the body mobilizes white blood cells to an area of toxicity where the cells will break down/digest toxins and dead tissues, preparing them for elimination, preferably outside of the bloodstream. If the inflammation is seen as the problem rather than the response and anti-inflammatory medications are given, the immune system is then forced to find a less efficient way of addressing the problem, perhaps resulting in chronic disease.

Normally, when toxins are eliminated from the blood, they will be eliminated through the skin in the form of a rash and/or via the mucous membranes in the form of a discharge. This "viral shedding" in diseases such as measles, rubella and chickenpox—even in the orthodox view—is acknowledged to be an important part of the resolution of illness and should not be suppressed.

A number of factors associated with an increased risk of suffering the paralytic form of polio would seem to bolster Beauchamp's view of disease. These include:

- exposure to DDT poisoning
- routine tonsillectomies
- removal of the appendix
- history of antibiotic use
- high exposure to sugar

In fact, in individuals whose tonsils had been removed (the fad surgery of the 1950s), there was a 700 percent increased risk of contracting paralytic polio. Perhaps we do benefit from *all* components of our immune system functioning! The allopathic approach to recurrent tonsillitis is to cut out the offending body part. A holistic approach to the same problem is to consider the underlying cause for recurrent infections and treat that.

Building the Immune System

Breastfeeding is undoubtedly the single most important proactive step mothers can take to build a strong immune system in their children. The immunities passed from mother to child through breastfeeding have long been acknowledged to be beneficial in all quarters. Despite recommendations from the AAP that favor exclusive breastfeeding for the first six months of life and continued breastfeeding to the age of two, only about 50 percent of U.S. babies are breastfed by six months of age. More recently, researchers studying Kangaroo Mother Care have discovered that *mothers who spend time skin-to-skin with their newborn infants are also passing immune factors to their babies via the skin.*

Secondly, it is important to avoid or minimize exposure to stresses that compromise the immune system. These include:

- unsanitary living conditions or overcrowding
- air and water pollution
- poor nutrition (especially over-indulgence in sugar and trans fats)
- overuse of alcohol, tobacco, marijuana, coffee, illicit drugs
- over-the-counter drugs (especially fever suppressors)
- steroids, cortisone creams, inhalers (steroids are designed to suppress the immune system, hence their use with organ transplant recipients so the patient will not reject the implanted foreign tissue)
- prescription drugs, antibiotics (see article on page 70, *Antibiotics: How Do They Harm Our Children)*
- stress
- inadequate sleep
- constipation, poor elimination of waste from the system

In addition, optimizing your family's nutritional status will go a long way towards reducing susceptibility to disease. The important role of essential fatty acids in the immune system is discussed in detail in the book by Leo Galland (see Resources). Using omega-3 oil supplements is recommended as most U.S. children are deficient in omega-3 fats. See also pages 75–7 for *Food & Herbal Sources of Important Immune System Nutrients.* My own book, *Whole Family Recipes—For the Childbearing Year & Beyond* (2007), focuses on simple strategies and delicious foods that support families as they transition to more healthful eating. New information on the importance of meat, animal fats and cholesterol (yes, cholesterol!) in the diet is also being published by the Weston A. Price Foundation. Going against conventional "wisdom" (including the "health food" movements of vegetarianism, macrobiotics, veganism, raw foods, etc.), Nancy Fallon argues for the importance of meat, animal fats and unpasteurized milk in her controversial book *Nourishing Traditions.*

Herbs and supplements can also be used to enhance the immune system and correct imbalances. See the *Family Winter Health Tea Recipe* (page 77), along with the article *Stimulating a Weakened Immune System* by Jane Sheppard (page 79).

Chiropractic care is yet another healing modality that can be used to enhance immune response. The nervous system controls functioning of all other body systems and organs. If nervous system functioning is optimized through chiropractic adjustment, immune system functioning is enhanced.

Finally, various forms of bodywork performed by a practitioner, or exercises that the individual undertakes himself, have been demonstrated to be helpful. Basically, any technique that increases circulation and movement of lymph through the nodes enhances the immune system. Possibilities include: massage, shiatsu, yoga, tai chi, chi kung and more. Even individuals whose mobility is limited or otherwise compromised, can benefit from massage or therapeutic yoga poses or perform the gentle chi kung exercises.

And let us not forget that true and lasting immunity from common childhood diseases can only be achieved by getting the disease. Perhaps it makes sense to simply not worry too much about healthy children over the age of one being exposed to measles, mumps, rubella and chickenpox. If they get these diseases as children, they will gain immunity from the more serious consequences when they are older and their immune systems will be encouraged to flower naturally, with minimal risk.

A Special Note on Fevers

Fever is a sign that the immune system is working. Body temperature rises in an effort to burn off invading viruses and bacteria. This is the body's natural defense system at work. The fever itself is not the problem; the underlying cause of the fever is the problem. *When fever suppressing medication is given, the immune system is hampered and the body responds less efficiently in its efforts to heal.* The result is the person may be sick for a longer period of time or be more prone to developing complications.

Much has been written about avoiding the use of aspirin with young children who have a fever due to the connection with the life-threatening Reyes Syndrome. It is my strong belief that Tylenol and other non-aspirin fever suppressors, while not life-threatening, should also be avoided whenever possible. Yes, your fever-stricken child will feel better temporarily if Tylenol is given. However supporting the body's path to healing itself calls for careful, close observance through the crisis (sleep next to the child) and frequent offering of fluids to avoid dehydration. Homeopathic remedies such as Belladonna, Aconite or others may be indicated for additional support to get you through the crisis and speed the body through its healing curve. (See page 85 for more information on homeopathy.)

Tylenol can still keep its place in the family medicine cabinet for its pain-relieving properties. Just remember, the fever is not the problem; it is part of the *solution.*

Antibiotics: How Do They Harm Our Children?

This article by Jane Sheppard is reprinted, with permission, from "Healthy Child ... a Publication of Future Generations," Volume 1, Number 2 (August/September, 1997) [http://healthychild.com]

Antibiotics are considered miracle drugs. They have saved many lives over the past 45 years. We are very fortunate to have them available to us for serious bacterial diseases. Unfortunately, antibiotics are now widely over-prescribed. There is an alarming, widespread, indiscriminate use of antibiotics in this country. This overuse of antibiotics can cause major health consequences.

In the book, *Beyond Antibiotics,* Drs. Michael Schmidt, Lendon Smith and Keith Sehnert explore the problems created by the overuse of antibiotics. They say that antibiotic misuse is most likely to occur in children under three years old. Ear infection, or *otitis media,* is the number one reason a child is brought to a doctor. Antibiotic therapy is the most common treatment for ear infections, with amoxicillin being the first choice of antibiotics by doctors in this country. The side effects of amoxicillin include upset stomach, diarrhea, allergic reactions and diaper rashes. The purpose of antibiotics is to kill harmful bacteria. Otitis media means middle ear inflammation—not infection. In many cases of otitis media (30 to 50 percent, according to *Beyond Antibiotics*), the middle ear contains no harmful bacteria. In a Dutch study of 2,975 children, it was found that 88 percent of children with acute otitis media never need antibiotics (Schmidt, *Childhood Ear Infections).* Other studies in the U.S. and Scandinavia came to similar conclusions.

The late Robert Mendelsohn, a highly respected pediatrician, wrote in his book *How to Raise a Healthy Child ... In Spite of Your Doctor,* "The only case in which the use of antibiotics can remotely be justified is if the ear is actually discharging pus, which occurs in less than one percent of ear infections and I'm not convinced that it can be justified even then."

I experienced indiscriminate use of antibiotics firsthand. When my daughter was about 13 months old, she had a fever of 104, was a little irritable, and had a clear runny nose. My mothering instincts and knowledge about teething told me that she was just cutting a new tooth. These symptoms can be present when a child is teething. I took her to her doctor anyway because of the high temperature. Her regular doctor was on vacation at the time and another doctor was filling in. She took a quick look in my daughter's ear, said it looked a little red, and started to write a prescription. I asked her what for and she told me she was prescribing an antibiotic; that it was protocol for an ear infection. I asked her why she thought there was a bacterial infection in my daughter's ear. She said she didn't know for sure, and the antibiotic was just to be on the safe side. I knew that teething can also cause middle ear redness and inflammation. I followed my instincts, refused the antibiotic, and gave my daughter a homeopathic teething remedy instead. By the next day, all her symptoms had disappeared and a molar had broken through my daughter's gums. In this case, the doctor had misdiagnosed common teething symptoms as an ear infection and tried to prescribe an antibiotic. Unfortunately, this scenario is quite common. Many parents unknowingly will accept the antibiotic, thinking that the doctor knows best.

Antibiotics fail to work in many cases and can actually worsen the health of a child. When a doctor prescribes antibiotics, the underlying reasons for the disease are usually ignored and left untreated. Antibiotics have also been shown to increase the likelihood of repeat infections.

Many children are dealing with a continuing cycle of repeat ear infections. A typical scenario is the child is diagnosed with acute otitis media and antibiotics are prescribed (whether a bacterial infection is present or not). The symptoms disappear in two weeks but return in another two weeks. The child goes back to the doctor for more antibiotics. The cycle continues. Some children spend months or even years on antibiotics, with recurring ear infections. Research has shown that when antibiotics are used at the beginning of an ear infection, the frequency of recurrence may be almost three times greater than if antibiotics are delayed or not used. The authors of *Beyond Antibiotics* point to evidence which suggests that antibiotics may limit the body's natural ability to identify and destroy invading bacteria. This may increase the likelihood of repeat infections.

Another reason for recurring infections is that antibiotics can cause a loss of nutrients in the body. Absorption of nutrients is also affected. Antibiotics adversely affect many nutrients, particularly the ones needed by the immune system to fight infections, such as vitamins A and C. One of the most common side effects of antibiotics is diarrhea. This causes a loss of nutrients, especially magnesium and zinc. Some children are on antibiotics for months or even years. Nutritional loss over such a long period of time is debilitating for the body and sets up an environment for more infections.

Beyond Antibiotics discusses the perils of antibiotic use. A very frightening consequence of indiscriminate use of antibiotics is the development of antibiotic-resistant bacteria. Because bacteria reproduce rapidly, they can quickly develop mutant offspring which are immune to antibiotics. This is becoming widespread. There are serious infectious diseases that are no longer responding to antibiotics. If an infection does respond, it often requires five to ten times the amount of the drug that used to be effective. Nearly every form of bacteria known to cause disease has been affected by antibiotic resistance.

Another problem with antibiotics is the destruction of the friendly bacteria, mainly in the intestinal tract. These bacteria are vital to good health. Among the more important bacteria are lactobacillus acidophilus and bifid bacterium bifidus. They help protect the body against infection. Antibiotics indiscriminately kill the beneficial as well as the "bad" bacteria. This can disrupt the balance of the intestines and lead to increased susceptibility to infections by fungi, bacteria, viruses and parasites.

When antibiotics are used excessively and beneficial bacteria are depleted, there may be an overgrowth of yeast in the body. Antibiotics can create a yeast infection which causes immune suppression which can also lead to recurrent infections.

Antibiotics can also cause allergic reactions. Sweeteners, dyes, flavorings and other unnamed additives are found in antibiotics. These may include saccharin, sucrose, red dye #40, FD & C yellow #5 and #6. These dyes are cross-reactive with aspirin and acetaminophen which are commonly given to a child during an illness. Even tiny amounts of the chemical additives in antibiotics can cause an allergic reaction in a sensitive child. It's important to always get a full disclosure of the contents of the drug being considered if your child has allergies or environmental sensitivity. Ask the pharmacist for the insert that comes with the medication.

Antibiotics are used by some doctors to treat the common cold or influenza which originate from viruses, not bacteria. This is clear misuse of antibiotics since they only kill bacteria and are of no value in treating viral infections. There are treatments that can relieve symptoms of a cold, but there is no drug (over-the-counter or prescription) that will cure a common cold. There is a private joke among doctors: without treatment a cold usually lasts about one week; with treatment it will last about seven days.

I want to emphasize that antibiotics may be absolutely necessary in certain situations, such as a life-threatening infection or when complications are present. We are very fortunate to have these drugs for appropriate situations. However, the authors of *Beyond Antibiotics* state emphatically that "Antibiotics should never be used alone. They should always be used in conjunction with methods that boost immunity and improve resistance."

Though written nearly two decades ago, the information in this article is very timely. In 2015, we are seeing the growth of antibiotic-resistant bacteria and related infections. According to the CDC, at least 2 million people per year suffer from antibiotic-resistant infections and, of those, approximately 23,000 per year die.

Food and Herbal Sources of Important Immune System Nutrients

Vitamin A   halibut liver oil, liver, cod liver oil, butter, egg yolk, carrots, apricots, sweet potatoes, green leafy vegetables, dandelion greens, alfalfa, parsley, yellow dock, capsicum, mallows

Vitamin B6   liver, milk products, Brewer's yeast, wheat germ/bran, kidney beans, sunflower seeds, soy products, bananas, molasses, cabbage, sunflower and sesame seeds, dandelion greens, watercress, wild mustard

Vitamin B9   liver, kidney, milk, Brewer's yeast, soy products, fresh nuts, wheat germ/bran, oats, unpolished rice, green leafy vegetables, ginseng

Vitamin C   raw fruits, tomatoes, green peppers, cabbage, brussel sprouts, broccoli, carrots, lettuce, rosehips, acerola, parsley,

	dandelion greens, watercress, plantain, mallows
Vitamin E	lamb's liver, eggs, herrings, wheat germ oil, soy products, leafy green vegetables, oatmeal, sunflower seeds, alfalfa, watercress
Copper	oysters, liver of young animals, Brewer's yeast, nuts and seeds, mushrooms, soy products, molasses, red clover, chickweed
Iron	liver, red meats, shellfish, eggs, rice polish, molasses, wheat germ, legumes, whole-grain cereals, dark green leafy vegetables, dried apricots, yeast, figs, dates, kelp, parsley, sunflower seeds, dandelion greens, alfalfa, sarsaparilla, yellow dock
Magnesium	seafood, milk, almonds, dates, walnuts, Brazil nuts, cashews, Brewer's yeast, green leafy vegetables, barley, soybeans, honey, kelp, alfalfa, lobelia, dandelion greens
Selenium	liver, eggs, fish, Brewer's yeast, wheat germ/bran, whole grains, brown rice, broccoli, tomatoes, cabbage, onions, garlic
Zinc	oysters, herrings, liver, wheat germ/bran, peas, whole nuts, carrots, green leafy

vegetables, yeast, broccoli, mushrooms, sunflower seeds, sprouted grains

Family Winter Health Tea Recipe

The following herbs are primarily nutritive in nature, providing much-needed vitamins and minerals in a form that the body can easily assimilate. The herbs also have an alkalinizing effect on the body. As the standard American diet is very acidic, the tea provides some balance. It is especially helpful for children who don't like vegetables or are otherwise fussy eaters. Most children don't need as much fruit juice as they may like to drink, as juice is very concentrated in sugars. Try diluting their juice with this tea and gradually get them accustomed to a less sweet taste (works best with non-acidic juices). There is no right or wrong way to make the tea. Play with it a bit, till you find a mixture that suits you and your children.

Ingredients

- Red Raspberry Leaves contain vitamins A, B, and E, as well as calcium, phosphorous, iron and an acid neutralizer.
- Nettles are a blood-cleansing and blood-building herb with a high iron content.
- Alfalfa contains vitamins A, D and E, as well as calcium and phosphorous.
- Rose Hips contain the entire vitamin C complex; good to boost the immune system.
- Spearmint is soothing to the stomach, aids in digestion and lends a pleasant taste to the mixture. A little goes a long way. (If you are taking homeopathic remedies, you should leave

the Spearmint out while the remedies are still active in your system as it is a known antidote.)
- Red Clover is a blood-purifying herb that can be added from time to time; especially recommended during acute illnesses.

Directions

Add a small handful of each herb to a one-gallon mason jar (or equivalent container); use a glass or other non-metal (aluminum is the worst) container with a lid. Cover the herbs with almost-boiling water and cap tightly. Steep this mixture from four to eight hours and then pour through a strainer and discard the herbs. The tea will stay fresh for about four days if kept in the refrigerator.

Purchasing Herbs

Herbs should be organic or wild-crafted. If the packaging doesn't say "organic" or "wild-crafted," it isn't. If you have these plants growing around you, try harvesting them yourself. Put them on a screen or hang them to dry and then store in an air-tight container, in a cool, dark place. Exposure to sunlight and temperature extremes (such as above the stove) will age your herbs more quickly. Dried herbs have a shelf life of one year if stored properly. Mail ordering herbs in higher quantities is the most cost-effective way to go, as the mark-up at your local health food store is likely to be significant. In addition, if your local store does not turn over herbs on a fairly regular basis, they may sit on the shelf too long and the quality will suffer, even to the point of molding.

Stimulating a Weakened Immune System

This article by Jane Sheppard is reprinted, with permission, from Healthy Child ... a Publication of Future Generations, Volume 1, Number 2 (August/September, 1997) [http://healthychild.com]

The amazing immune system, your child's natural defense against disease, is constantly working to keep your child healthy. It can sometimes become weakened though, due to a number of factors. These factors include diet, excessive antibiotic use, formula feeding, vaccination, emotional stress, genetics, environmental pollutants and physical/spinal trauma. Emphasis needs to be placed on boosting immunity with healing modalities that treat the whole child, rather than treating the sickness.

The first issue of *Healthy Child* discussed building and maintaining a healthy immune system with nutritional foods, breastfeeding and paying attention to emotional health. It's important to take a look at diet, food allergies, environmental pollutants, toxins and emotional stress as possible causes of weakened immunity. The cause needs to be addressed first. This article will provide ways to boost immunity through supplementation and other forms of healing. There are excellent healing modalities available for dealing with suppressed immunity that have not been included in this article, but are certainly options to consider. These include chiropractic, therapeutic massage, hands-on-healing, acupuncture and oriental medicine, as well as different aspects of emotional healing. There is too much information to cover on these topics to be included here, but they will be covered in detail in future issues of *Healthy Child.*

Nutritional Supplements

Nutritional deficiencies may be responsible for chronic immune problems, since it's easier for bacteria or viruses to take hold when important nutrients are missing. Chronic infections can also affect nutrition by impairing appetite and absorption. In addition, when a child is sick, the body uses its store of nutrients faster than usual. You may want to consult a health professional who knows a lot about nutrition to find out if your child has any deficiencies. Good nutrition is vital to the immune system. Flaxseed oil (essential fatty acids) and antioxidant nutrients such as vitamins A, C, E, zinc and selenium can be used to supplement your child's diet. Keep in mind that high doses of zinc (over 100 mg) can *suppress* immunity.

When your child begins to show signs of a cold or infection, vitamin C may be able to prevent it from taking hold. According to Lendon Smith, M.D., in *Feed Your Kids Right,* vitamin C can be taken every one to two hours at the following age-adjusted doses: 50 to 100 mg for infants under 6 months old; 100 to 200 mg for infants 6 to 12 months old; 500 mg for kids 1 to 5 years old; and 1,000 mg for kids 6 and over. The concept of bowel tolerance has also been used to find the right dose. The intent is to increase the dose until the stools become loose; then decrease the dose gradually until the stools become normal. This is the optimal dose. There is no toxicity associated with high doses of vitamin C. It has been studied extensively and found to have a very wide margin of safety.

The authors of *Beyond Antibiotics* suggest that vitamin C be taken during and after an infection. Bioflavonoids are necessary to enhance the activity of vitamin C. They stimulate immune function and are naturally found in the foods that contain vitamin C. Powdered vitamin C is more efficiently utilized than tablets. You can find powdered vitamin C with bioflavonoids in most health food stores. Ascorbic acid has been shown to dissolve tooth enamel so teeth need to be brushed afterward if using chewable vitamin C.

If your child has been taking antibiotics, the beneficial bacteria of his/her intestinal tract may also be eliminated in the process. These bacteria are extremely important to the health of your child. The "good" bacteria need to be replenished. The beneficial bacteria supplements are called probiotics. You may want to consider probiotic supplementation if your child has a history of antibiotic use, ear infections, oral thrush, diarrhea, constipation, colic, food allergies, eczema, intestinal viral infections or candidiasis, or is bottle-fed.

Yogurt contains two main species of the beneficial bacteria, but in this form they are unable to attach to the intestinal wall and establish themselves permanently in the intestines. Therefore, the healing effects of yogurt do not last long.

Acidophilus is the probiotic supplement suggested for children over seven and bifidus for children under seven. In his book, *Childhood Ear Infections,* Dr. Michael A. Schmidt gives guidelines for buying these supplements. He suggests purchasing a powdered product that is refrigerated at all times. The label should state the number of viable organisms. There should be at least one billion or more. It should also state the identifiable strain. The strains that have been thoroughly tested are DDS1 and NCFM. Enteric coating is not necessary and could interfere with maximum release of the bacteria. Dr. Schmidt also maintains that the most viable strains of acidophilus and bifidus are only able to live in a dairy base. They need calcium to attach to the intestinal wall and colonize. They are grown on milk solids, and then the milk solids are filtered off, leaving only a small amount of the dairy substrate. This minimizes the chance of a dairy-allergic child reacting. If your child is vegan, nondairy products are also available.

Dr. Schmidt recommends taking ¼ teaspoon of powder in ¼ glass of lukewarm water to begin supplementation. Dosage is often increased to ½ or 1 full teaspoon one to three times daily. Or follow your own health practitioner's recommendations. The supplements should be taken during mid-meal.

Essential Oils

There has been extensive research in Europe in the use of essential oils (plant oils) for treatment of infections. It's been shown that plant oils interfere with the bacteria's ability to breathe. Some oils boost immunity and some are directly bactericidal, fungicidal and veridical. They are easily absorbed through the skin into the bloodstream. They can also be inhaled.

Lavender oil has been studied extensively and is known to boost immunity. It can be rubbed into your child's skin to help prevent illness. A massage with lavender oil can be a wonderfully healing experience for your child. Remember that massage can also boost the immune system.

Another way to protect your child from contagious diseases is to add a few drops of eucalyptus *radiata* or tea tree oil to his/her bathwater. Make sure you are using pure essential oils. In addition, six to eight drops of eucalyptus *radiata* oil in a diffuser or warm-air vaporizer will cleanse and purify the air while your child is sleeping.

A gentle massage can be very comforting to a child with flu or chest cold. Massage should be avoided if high fever is present. A massage oil made from 2 drops of lavender oil, 1 to 2 drops eucalyptus oil, and 2 drops chamomile oil added to 1 ounce carrier oil can be rubbed on the chest, moving from the middle of the chest out toward the armpit. This can relieve discomfort, loosen mucus and fight infection. Lavender and tea tree oils are both excellent antiseptics for cuts or burns. Tea tree oil is antibacterial and antifungal.

Herbal Therapy
The herb echinacea is widely used to stimulate a weakened immune system. There are over 350 scientific studies of echinacea. It is being used internally to combat viruses and bacteria as well as externally for healing wounds. It's been shown to kill yeast and fight inflammation. Echinacea has been used for hundreds of years with no toxic side effects. Research shows it is very safe for children, except for a possibility of a rare allergic reaction in someone who is extremely sensitive. Children's echinacea tinctures are nonalcoholic and taste good. They can be found at your local health food store. If you are nursing, your child will receive the echinacea you take through your breast milk.

Chinese astragalus root is a good tonic herb that has been used for thousands of years to stimulate the immune system and to fight disease. It can be used long-term, although it should be avoided in high fever situations, since it is a heat-producing herb.

Garlic is an excellent immune booster. It is a powerful antiviral, antifungal and antibacterial herb. It's been shown to be more effective than penicillin for sore throats. It's been studied extensively and found to be effective in treating many types of infection, including yeast overgrowth. It can be served raw in salad dressing, guacamole or veggie dip or added at the last minute to soups, etc. Cooking destroys some of its active ingredients and minimizes the antibiotic affects. You can make garlic-veggie juice by adding 1–3 cloves to 8 oz. fresh vegetable juice. You can also make garlic-honey cough syrup. A small clove or (1/2) can be swallowed with water by an older child if there is no danger of choking. You can also get it in capsules or tablets, although most deodorized garlic has little direct antibiotic effect.

Ginger, garlic, nettles and cayenne are all herbs with immune-stimulating properties that can be added to your child's food as much as possible. Kelp powder can be used instead of salt. Kelp is a good balanced mineral food for the immune system.

THE ROLE OF HOMEOPATHY

Introduction to Homeopathy

Homeopathy is a 200+ year-old system of safe and effective holistic treatment that is practiced worldwide. It is well-suited to home health care for first aid and acute illness and does not carry the risks associated with drug treatments. Constitutional treatment can cure chronic tendencies to illness and prevent relapses (i.e., recurrent ear infections), as well as eliminate a genetically-determined predisposition for certain weaknesses or diseases (known as *miasms)*. Constitutional treatment is most successful when overseen by an experienced homeopath. See the National Center for Homeopathy (see Resources) for help in finding a reputable, *classical homeopath* near you. Some classical homeopaths have begun to treat patients via Skype as well, if that is your only option.

Homeopathy is non-toxic, free of side-effects (for the most part) and safe. The worst that critics allege is (1) that homeopathic pellets get their results from the placebo effect and (2) that a delay in procuring urgent medical care for a person in crisis may occur while one attempts to self-medicate.

Since homeopathy brings relief to infants, animals and those in a state of unconsciousness, as well as demonstrating superior outcomes in double-blind, controlled clinical trials [http://hpathy.com/scientific-research/database-of-positive-homeopathy-research-studies/], we can dismiss the placebo-effect allegation. The second point regarding delays in seeking needed medical care is a good one. With that caveat in mind, we need not take an all-or-nothing approach. One can pursue standard medical care and use homeopathic remedies simultaneously. It is possible that, by the time one arrives at the hospital, the remedies will have made the trip to the ER moot. So much the better. Rather than suppressing symptoms with potentially toxic medications, the goal is to allow the disease to run its course while supporting efficient functioning of the immune system and preventing serious complications. Typically, when homeopathic treatment is used, the overall course of an illness is shortened.

Historically, homeopathy has effected impressive successes in the disease epidemics of the 1800s, including cholera, typhoid and scarlet fever. Mortality rates in homeopathic hospitals were significantly lower than in conventional hospitals. For example, during the cholera epidemic in England in 1855, with conventional treatment, mortality was 51.9 percent; with homeopathic treatment, the mortality rate was 16.3 percent. Likewise, during a cholera epidemic in Cincinnati in 1849, the mortality rate with homeopathic treatment was 3 percent whereas, with conventional treatment, mortality rates ranged from 40–70 percent.

How does homeopathy work? There are two central concepts to this 200-plus-year-old system of medicine. The first is known as the *Law of Similars.* The idea that *a substance can cure symptoms in a sick person similar to those that it causes in a healthy person* was written about by Hypocrites, Paracelsus and Frances Bacon, and even appeared in the Hindu system of Ayurvedic medicine as far back as the tenth century B.C. The concept was rediscovered by eighteenth century German physician Samuel Hahnemann who found that the reason quinine cured malaria was because it was capable of causing the symptoms of malaria in a healthy person. Hence the name, "homeo" (similar) + "pathy" (suffering). Hahnemann went on to experiment with numerous natural substances, expanding the applications of this healing principle. The homeopathic pharmacopoeia today consists of over 2,000 medicines, called *remedies*. These remedies come primarily from plant, animal and mineral sources.

The second key concept is known as the *Law of Potentization.* This law refers to the pharmaceutical process that renders a natural substance into a homeopathic remedy. While applying the *Law of Similars,* Hahnemann began to experiment with the concept of the *minimum dose* of a substance required to activate a healing response. The minimum dose, he reasoned, would reduce the occurrence of unwanted drug effects or "side effects." In a way that modern physics cannot yet fully explain, the process of potentization—serial dilution of a full strength extract, followed by succussion or rapid shaking after each dilution—activates dormant energy in matter. This dynamic, or non-material dose is thought to impart the vibrational imprint of the plant or other substance by way of the body's *vital force,* thereby stimulating a healing response. The number/letter combinations noted after the remedy name (e.g., 6X, 30C, 1M), indicate the potency or strength of the remedy.

Treatment with homeopathy consists of close observation of the unique symptom picture expressed by the individual patient and then matching their symptoms with a remedy capable of producing a similar set of symptoms in a healthy person.

In the context of our current discussion on the vaccine issue, what is the role of homeopathy? The following applications are discussed: (1) remedies that can be given prior to and immediately after vaccination in order to neutralize the shock to the system, hopefully mitigating, or preventing altogether, adverse vaccine reactions; (2) remedies that can be used to treat adverse reactions to vaccines if they occur, including suspected long-term effects, known as "constitutional" treatment; (3) remedies that can be given prophylactically, after exposure to an infectious disease, to prevent infection; (4) remedies that can be used to treat infection if it does occur, mitigate the severity of the disease, shorten the duration considerably, prevent complications and clear up lingering after-effects; and (5) a controversial prophylactic routine of remedy administration, known as "homeopathic vaccination."

What follows is a compilation of recommendations from homeopathic authors listed in the Resources. Ideally, it is recommended that you consult a homeopathic physician who can "take the case," choose a remedy for your child, and make recommendations regarding dosage, while following your child through the course of the illness back to a state of health. However, I am well aware that competent and affordable homeopathic assistance is a luxury that not everyone can easily access in the U.S. Due to this limitation, I have long believed in making homeopathy as accessible as possible for all and encouraging its use by homeopathic moms and dads in the home.

Please keep the following points in mind:

- Where more than one remedy is listed for prophylaxis, the one listed first and marked with an asterisk is most frequently recommended in the literature and should be your first choice, if available.

- Many of the prophylactic remedies listed belong to a special category of remedies known as *nosodes* (a homeopathic remedy made from diseased tissue or morbid matter). Nosodes are not as readily available to consumers without a prescription. You might develop your own sources for these remedies, but if you can't access them, use the non-nosode remedy listed.

- In each treatment section, the remedies listed are those most frequently mentioned in the literature as being helpful in treating these diseases and should be considered first to see if they are a match for the patient's symptoms.

- The prophylactic remedies listed may also be indicated during the course of the illness itself or afterwards, for lingering effects. Unless I had specific recommendations to pass on, I didn't double-list them in the treatment sections.

- It is not my intention to provide sufficient information here to select an appropriate remedy if your child suffers a serious vaccine reaction or gets the disease. Rather, I am attempting to narrow down the selection for the home prescriber and am presuming that you have the capacity to consult other, more detailed and authoritative sources (see Resources).

- For a brief *materia medica* (description of a remedy's symptom picture) of the remedies listed, see the Boericke and/or Morrison books listed in the Resources. Dorothy Shepherd's *Homoeopathy in Epidemic Diseases* contains invaluable advice, based on years of clinical experience treating these diseases, as well as symptom pictures of the remedies listed. In addition, you will find that many of the introductory books on homeopathy for family health care contain recommendations for measles, mumps, chickenpox, influenza and tetanus.

- It is important to note that during the course of an illness, as the symptom picture changes, a different remedy may be indicated.

- *Finally, do not hesitate to seek allopathic medical care for any condition discussed as some may be life threatening. Homeopathic treatment can still be pursued congruently and will not interact with other medications, since it is working on an energetic level in the body rather than saturating the bloodstream with medicinal agents.*

Homeopathy and Vaccine Reactions

Routine Prophylaxis for Vaccine Reactions

Ledum 30C—3 doses per day for 1 day prior and 3 days after vaccination
and
Hypericum 30C—same dosage as above, take concurrently with Ledum
and
Thuja 30C—3 doses, 12 hours apart, after live virus vaccines

Treating Acute Reactions
Try 3–4 doses, over 24 hours, in 30C potency or 1–2
doses in 200C of one of the following remedies.

Apis — allergic reaction, arm swells, hives, itching, fever, thirstless, symptoms worse from heat and better from cold

Belladonna — arm swells up, is red and hot to touch, throbbing sensation, fever, symptoms worse from jarring

Hypericum — sharp radiating pain or shooting pain from the injection site

Ledum — sore, achy, bruised, red streaks, cold to touch, injection site doesn't heal well

Pulsatilla — after MMR or DTaP, #1 remedy for infectious childhood diseases (and related vaccines); give if you are unsure what to give, or if other chosen remedies fail

Stramonium — febrile states, delirious, seizures; after neurological insult such as vaccination

If Infection is Present
Dosage same as above, but higher potencies may also
be indicated.

Echinacea | septicemia (blood infection), high fever, sweat, offensive breath, achy muscles

Hepar Sulph | local abscess with pus, whole arm painful, hypersensitive to touch, symptoms worse from cold and better from warmth

Pyrogenium | systemic infection, fast pulse/low fever or slow pulse/high fever, injection site never heals, offensiveness, restless and better from motion, aching through whole body, sore and bruised feeling, bed feels too hard, delirium, throbbing headache; good general antidote for multiple vaccinations

Treating Chronic Reactions

Homeopaths see vaccines as an etiology for a lot of health problems, especially neurological symptoms and diseases of the mucous membranes. Chronic problems are best treated with the help of an experienced homeopath. Some homeopaths will use one dose of a high potency, while others may recommend low doses repeated.

Silica | most often indicated, especially for infants; lost vitality, weakened by the vaccine; respiratory problems and tendency for colds

Thuja	used historically for after-effects of the smallpox vaccine; asthma; skin problems such as acne, cysts, eczema, warts; good general antidote for animal poisons
Pulsatilla	"Never well since" MMR or DTaP
Vaccine Nosode	one dose daily of 30C until better or one dose of 200C or 1M; these are potentized versions of the vaccines, e.g., MMR nosode; see above for information on nosodes and their availability

Homeopathic Prophylaxis and Treatment of Infectious Childhood Diseases

Chickenpox

Prophylaxis: *You may want to let your children get chickenpox and get it over with. Prevent in newborns.*

*Antimonium tart 30—one dose daily after exposure for 14 days

Varicella 30 (nosode)—one dose every four hours for three doses; then once weekly while there is risk of infection

Malandrinum 30—dosage as for
Antimonium tart above

Treatment: *Suppression of the skin eruptions with
anti-viral drugs (acyclovir) is not
recommended. Try calamine lotion on the
itching lesions and/or soak the child in
aveeno baths (avoid versions of these
products containing camphor which is
known to antidote homeopathic
remedies).*

#1 remedy is Rhus tox
#2 remedy is Antimonium crudum

Mercurius viv, Pulsatilla, Rhus tox,
Sulphur

Diphtheria

Prophylaxis: *Should be prevented as it is a severe
disease, especially in children under the
age of 5.*

*Diphtherinum 30 (nosode)—once per
week for 4–6 weeks during risk of
infection or one dose every four hours for
three doses followed by one dose weekly
while there is risk of infection (4-6
weeks)

Pyrogen 30 (nosode)—dosage choices
same as above

Apis 30 (if nosodes are unavailable)—
dosage choices same as above

Treatment: Arsenicum, Lac caninum, Lachesis,
Mercurius cyanatus, Phytolacca,
Gelsemium (for after effects, i.e., post-
diphtheritic paralysis when fluids
regurgitate through the nose)

Haemophilus Influenza Type B (HIB)

Prophylaxis: *This disease should be prevented. Most*
susceptible group is between the ages of
6 months and 4 years, with an increased
risk (up to 50 percent) for children in
large daycare settings.

Meningococcus 30 (nosode)—one dose
in the morning three times per week for
two weeks following contact with the
disease

and
Belladonna 30—one dose in the evening
three times per week for two weeks
following contact with the disease

Treatment: Gelsemium, Natrum Sulph

Hepatitis B

Prophylaxis: This disease should be prevented.

Hepatitis B 30 (nosode)—three doses 12 hours apart following a high-risk incident such as dubious injection or operation

Chelidonium—5 drops of mother tincture in water three times per day or one dose per day of 6X while at risk

Treatment: Lycopodium, Natrum Sulph, Phosphorus

Influenza

During the influenza epidemic of 1918–20, the overall mortality rate was 30 percent; 25,000 Americans died. With homeopathic treatment, the mortality rate was 1 percent.

Prophylaxis: Influenzinum 30 (nosode)—one dose three times a week during an epidemic or one dose night and morning for three days; then once weekly while at risk

Aconite, Gelsemium and Eupatorium 30 (combination)—one dose every twelve hours for three days following contact with the disease; more frequently if symptoms develop

Tuberculinum 30 (nosode)—to prevent recurrent attacks, especially for influenza that goes into the lungs; one dose per month from October through March

Treatment: Give indicated remedy in 30C potency, diluted in water, every 2 hours or so at the onset, then go to every 4 hours

Arsenicum, Bryonia, Eupatorium, Gelsemium, Influenzinum ("never well since"), Rhus tox

Measles

Prophylaxis: *Highly contagious; may want to let children get it and get it over with. Most dangerous in children under 5 years old.*

Pulsatilla 30—once daily for 15–16 days after exposure or once weekly during epidemic without direct exposure

Morbillinum 30 (nosode)—once weekly for 2 weeks after contact

Treatment: Pulsatilla—#1 all-round measles remedy; excellent post-measles remedy

Belladonna, Bryonia, Euphrasia, Gelsemium, Morbillinum (for lingering severe cases with weight loss and debility; to prevent lung complications), Rhus tox, Sulphur

Mumps

Prophylaxis: *May want to let children get mumps, if exposed. Should be prevented in adult males.*

*Pilocarpine 30—one dose per day for 10–12 days after exposure

Parotidinum 30 (nosode)—one dose per week for two weeks following contact with the disease

Trifolium repens 30—one dose per day for 10–12 days after exposure

Treatment: Pilocarpine—#1 remedy for acute mumps; 2 doses daily for 3 days; for after-effects, twice daily for 3–5 days

*Parotidinum—night & morning from onset for 5 days; or for after-effects, "never well since"

Apis, Belladonna, Jaborandi, Lycopodium, Mercurius viv, Phytolacca, Pulsatilla

Pertussis (Whooping Cough)

Prophylaxis: *Should be prevented as it is a severe disease. Especially important to prevent in infants under the age of 1. Prevent people coughing near babies. Children under the age of 5 are at greater risk generally. See Dr. Dorothy Shepherd's account of the efficacy of homeopathic prevention and treatment of whooping cough in* <u>Homeopathy in Epidemic Diseases</u>*.*

*Pertussin 30 (nosode)—once daily for 2 weeks after exposure, or once per week during an epidemic, or if person is already beginning the catarrhal stage, then 3–4 times daily to prevent paroxysmal stage

Drosera 30 (if nosode is unavailable)—dosage as above

Treatment: *Antibiotics are often prescribed for pertussis, but they have minimal effect on symptoms. Antibiotics do kill the bacterium that causes pertussis and may prevent spread of the disease to others. Cough suppressants are useless.*

#1 remedy is Drosera
#2 remedy is Cuprum metallicum

Carbo vegetabilis, Coccus cacti, Ipecac

Polio

Prophylaxis: *Not a highly-contagious disease, but can have severe complications. Should be prevented. Children under the age of five are especially susceptible.*

*Lathyrus sativus 30—one dose per week for three weeks following any contact with the disease or during epidemic

Poliomyelitis 30 (nosode)—dosage same as above

Gelsemium 30—dosage same as above

Treatment: *The three remedies listed for prophylaxis are the top treatment remedies as well.*

Rubella (German Measles)

Prophylaxis: *Prevent in pregnant women. Otherwise, you may want to let your children get rubella and get it over with in order to gain life-long immunity.*

*Pulsatilla 30—one dose daily for 10-14 days after exposure or once monthly if pregnant and not immune

Rubella 30 (nosode)—one dose 3 times per week for 3 weeks after exposure

Treatment: Belladonna, Mercurius

Tetanus

Prophylaxis: *This life-threatening disease is important to prevent. Get puncture wounds to bleed, clean them well with antiseptic and irrigate with sterile saline solution. See discussion on tetanus (pages 47–9) and remember, tetanus immune globulin can be given to unvaccinated or under-vaccinated people (meaning those with less than two previous doses of the toxoid vaccine) who have suffered high-risk or moderate-risk injuries.*

Hypericum (or Ledum) tincture—diluted 1 part tincture to 9 parts water, to cleanse the wound *(Warning: do not use Calendula preparations on puncture wounds; it may speed healing of outer layers too quickly and actually seal in infection.)*

and
*Ledum 30—3–4 doses daily for several days for puncture wounds or animal bites

and/or
Hypericum 30—3–4 doses daily for contaminated wounds that are not punctures or any wound with upward shooting pain from the site of an injury

Clostridium tetani 30 (nosode)—one dose per week during high-risk activities (i.e., trekking, mountaineering, exploring) or one dose twice per week for three weeks following injury

Treatment: *If signs of infection develop such as increased pain, redness and swelling, seek medical help.*

*Hypericum 30 or 200 (if signs of infection are present)

Homeopathic "Vaccines"

The use of homeopathic vaccines (giving a course of remedies at regular intervals, similar to vaccines, as a disease prevention strategy) is controversial, even within the homeopathic community. Dr. Isaac Golden discusses the controversy and history of their use. If you are interested in looking into this possibility, I suggest that you purchase his book, *Vaccination & Homoeoprophylaxis? A Review of Risks and Alternatives,* 7th Edition (2010).

CLAIMING AN EXEMPTION

When Are Waivers Required?
Vaccine waiver forms are used in situations where proof of vaccination must be submitted in order for your child to participate. These mandates apply to children attending licensed daycare, public or private school, most summer camps, and most colleges and universities.

General Recommendations
- *Know your rights.* If you do not know them, you may as well not have them because you will be at the mercy of what others believe and say.
- *Know the exact wording of the law in your state,* which can be found here: http://www.nvic.org/vaccine-laws/state-vaccine-requirements.aspx.

Medical Exemptions
Medical exemptions are typically signed by a medical doctor and are based on contraindications listed in vaccine package inserts. Medical exemptions are considered temporary so parents may have to repeatedly find a doctor to sign off on this exemption, even if their child has a long-term disability that contraindicates vaccination.

Religious Exemptions

Some states require that you be an "adherent" or "member" of a recognized church whose teachings are opposed to vaccination (e.g., Christian Science Church, Universal Life Church, etc.). Other states require only that you hold "bonafide" or "sincere" religious beliefs opposed to vaccines. Such beliefs may or may not include belief in God or the scriptures. To be "sincere," beliefs must be central in importance in a person's life and the person must be living according to these beliefs.

Philosophical/Other Exemptions

Check the wording of your state law. Philosophical exemptions may be described variously as good cause, parental objection, personal or moral convictions, conscientiously held beliefs, etc. When claiming this exemption, use the exact wording of your state law. It is not necessary to go into the reasons for your choice.

Strategies/Considerations

If there is a possibility that you may move out of state (or your child may one day attend college in another state), you may want to develop a legal strategy that will demonstrate consistency in your position regarding exemptions. If you ever end up in court, inconsistency in your claim will most likely work against you. Consider, for example, that while some states have religious, philosophical or other exemptions, many other states do not. Switching from a philosophical exemption to a religious one could be problematic in terms of demonstrating consistency. Furthermore, doing away with religious and philosophical exemptions is often a priority for pro-vaccine forces when proposing new legislation. Organized consumer efforts are necessary to ensure that such restrictive legislation does not pass.

Exceptions/Limitations on Exemptions

- Privately-funded schools may refuse to allow exemptions. All schools that receive state aid and come under the jurisdiction of the Health Department have provisions for exemptions. A good way to find out whether or not a daycare provider receives state aid is to ask whether or not they participate in the government lunch program. If so, then they must accept exemptions according to state law.
- Most states have tied vaccine compliance to welfare benefits.
- The law allows schools to refuse your child admittance during outbreaks of vaccine-preventable diseases. However, proof of immunity, through a doctor's statement or a blood test, can be submitted to keep your child in school.

If Your Exemption is Denied

- If denied, get it in writing.
- Find out the reason for the denial and resubmit your request.
- If still denied, go above the person's head who denied you (to the principal, the school superintendent, the school board).
- Document all conversations and phone calls.

- Call the NVIC for a referral to an attorney who specializes in vaccine law (see Resources).

Dealing with Coercion

Neil Miller's book, *Immunization Theory vs. Reality,* contains a summary of tactics used to coerce people into vaccinating their children. I think it can be very helpful for parents who find themselves on the defensive, to understand that what they are experiencing is not personal, but rather part of larger pattern, even policy of coercion. Here is a sampling of Miller's suggestions for dealing with pressure from outsiders:

- "My children are taken care of in that department."
- "Yes, I will see that they will be protected."
- At the pediatrician's office: "Not at this time."
- If confronted by emergency room personnel: Ask for the release form.

Remember that you are not obligated to discuss your vaccination decision with anyone. Often parents are met with closed-minded arrogance and judgment if they are making a choice outside of the norm. It may be in your best interest to simply insist upon your rights to make a choice, rather than on all the reasons for the choice, and to otherwise be evasive. You don't *owe* anyone an explanation (and this includes extended family members as well).

For example, earlier this year, Michigan passed legislation requiring parents seeking waivers to attend an "educational session" at their local public health department. On the Michigan Opposing Mandatory

Vaccines (MOM) Facebook forum, there seems to be much trepidation expressed around upcoming health department visits to obtain exemptions. While I can understand annoyance at the required visit, some parents appear to fundamentally misunderstand the nature of this requirement. When claiming legal waivers, parents are acting within the law while, on the other hand, public health employees are simply doing their job. It is not necessary to convince anyone of the reasons for your choices. My advice is to stay calm and respectful and, if you must express your anger, save it for the legislators who passed the restrictive legislation. For example, one can simply say "I prefer not to discuss my reasons with you. I am here to claim my legal right to an exemption in accordance with state law."

It is worth noting here, that the form provided by the state of Michigan contains the following language:

> *"By signing this waiver, I acknowledge that I have been informed that I may be placing my child and others at risk of serious illness should she or he contract a disease that could have been prevented through proper vaccination."*

A number of strategies have been attempted by parents completing this waiver. In the past, some parents have substituted a waiver form of their own provided by MOM. Others have crossed out this one line before signing and submitting the form. And still others have attempted to indicate that they are signing "under duress" on the form. It is very likely that, under the new law, officials may no longer accept any alterations to the exemption claim form. It still may be possible to indicate duress by inserting "V.C." (Latin for "vis compulsiva," which translates as "compulsive force") *before your signature* and without comment. This may go unchallenged and serve to indicate your disagreement with the process. Since each state is different, parents will need to do a bit of research before proceeding with the claim process.

To gain a better understanding of the strategies used against anyone questioning the safety or wisdom of mass vaccination, read "First They Came for the Anti-Vaxxers" by Bretigne Shaffer (a blog published on LewRockwell.com, April 23, 2015). This is an excellent, well-referenced summary of how the media handles vaccine-related stories. Shaffer identifies ten key strategies of the media's "vaccine playbook." I highly recommend reading the full article for the commentary and citations that accompany each of the playbook strategies. Following is a brief summary of the strategies (recognize any?):

1. *Make it clear that parents who choose not to vaccinate their children are only getting their information from celebrities with absolutely no scientific credentials.*

2. *Always equate the views of the CDC, medical journals and pharmaceutical company spokespeople with "science."*

3. *Remind your readers that, however heart wrenching or tragic, anecdotal accounts are just that.*

4. *Remind your readers that "correlation is not causation."*

5. *Whenever possible, present the debate as if there are no legitimate reasons to choose not to*

vaccinate—only "personal beliefs" and "irrational fears."

6. *If you must acknowledge that critics of vaccines have actual reasons for their concerns, restrict the discussion to the fear that vaccines may cause autism and be sure to stress that the only basis for this concern is the retracted 1998 study by Andrew Wakefield.*

7. *Pepper your stories with the following affirmations: "Vaccines save lives," "parents who don't vaccinate are selfish" ("ignorant" and "anti-science" work well too), and "the science is settled."*

8. *Don't even address vaccines directly. Simply mention that vaccine skepticism is an example of the kind of irrational thinking some people still engage in despite "everyone knowing" how foolish it is.*

9. *If the icky topic of conflict of interest or corruption of the research by vested interests comes up, just laugh it off.*

10. *Remind your readers of our long-treasured right to herd immunity—to demand that others take every possible precaution against contracting communicable diseases, regardless of the risks to themselves of doing so.*

Source:
[https://www.lewrockwell.com/2015/04/bretigne-shaffer/first-they-came-for-the-anti-vaxxers/]

Vigilance is the Price of Freedom
It seems that at regular intervals, pro-vaccine forces are eager to take away parents' right to choose. After an

outbreak of measles in California this past winter, opposition to parental rights in the matter of vaccine choice became headline national news and it is coming from both ends of the political spectrum. Please consider supporting the NVIC (see Resources). Under the leadership of Barbara Loe Fisher, the NVIC has been fighting effectively for decades to make vaccines safer and to protect a citizen's right to choose whether or not to vaccinate. Check also to see if there is a vaccine consumer group active in your state. These groups make it their business to pay close attention to proposed vaccine-related legislation, monitor legislators' voting records and keeps members informed with newsletters, timely updates and legislative action alerts. Facebook forums of like-minded parents in your state can be another great way of staying in the information flow.

Finding a Doctor Who Supports Parental Choice

For parents whose choice is to avoid all vaccines, or to give some vaccines and not others, or to alter the vaccine schedule in any way, it can often be a challenge to find a willing pediatrician to provide health care for your child. I have heard reports ranging from relentless harassment at every doctor's office visit to refusal to accept you as a patient if you refuse to comply. Check the Sears' website for a directory of "vaccine-friendly" doctors [http://www.askdrsears.com/topics/health-concerns/vaccines/find-vaccine-friendly-doctor-near-you]. And, if you don't find what you are looking for there, contact the consumer group in your state or local Facebook forums for help in identifying health care providers who support parental choice.

You may not find a flexible or holistic pediatrician per se, but perhaps there is a family practice doctor willing to support you. See also *How to Raise a Healthy Child in Spite of your Doctor* by Robert Mendelsohn, MD for an insider's critique of the pediatric profession. He explains how "well-baby check-ups" came about as a means to enable vaccination. Mendelsohn claims that the practice of taking healthy babies to doctors is simply not necessary and was instituted by the profession to generate income. If you choose, you can simply sidestep these regular check-ups where you will be pressured to vaccinate and thereby also limit your child's exposure to other sick children. Unless you have a sick infant who requires the care of a pediatric specialist, a family practice doctor should be able to provide competent care for the entire family, including newborns and infants.

IN CONCLUSION

Clearly, vaccination is a complicated and controversial issue. It is my belief that there is not one right answer for everybody. Each family must undertake their own unique risk assessment, as well as balancing a complex array of other considerations including health factors, religious beliefs, lifestyle choices and socio-economic constraints. For example, some folks live on horse farms, some must rely on daycare for their child and others may be planning travel to Third World countries. It can be very challenging to resolve all concerns to both parents' satisfaction and compromise may be called for.

In my work over the years with hundreds of childbearing couples, I have repeatedly come up against one phenomenon that I would like to address. And that is the issue of *fear*. The germ paradigm promotes the idea that disease is out there to get us. This mentality preys on fear and creates more fear—fear of diseases lurking everywhere, fear of the vaccines, fear of the government, fear of the pediatrician's response, fear of family and social pressure, and so on.

The materials in this book have been gathered to encourage informed decision-making based on knowledge of alternatives. Alternatives include every proactive step you can take to: (1) build your child's immune system; (2) employ a holistic approach to disease and disease prevention; and (3) keep your legal options open. There is a great deal that is within your power, but you will be exactly as powerless as you believe yourself to be. A decision to comply with vaccine recommendations is made safer by an informed consumer who is taking precautions to avoid adverse reactions and who understands her/his rights. There is no doubt that whatever your choice, if you are reading this book, you are endeavoring to make an informed one. You should then rest easy in the knowledge that you are behaving conscientiously and doing what you believe is best for your child. That is all any of us can reasonably do. The concepts of reducing individual susceptibility to disease and taking personal responsibility for our health are the most empowering pathways out of fear.

We live in a society that *encourages* an irrational fear of disease and this fear, fueled by greed, ignorance and a compliant media, creates an atmosphere wherein mass brainwashing is possible and we are its victims. If you choose to step outside of this dynamic and apply reason to the problem, you may find that you are unique in your family or school, but *you are not alone.* A growing number of informed and concerned parents are asking questions and entertaining reservations regarding vaccines. After careful consideration, I urge you to trust yourself to make the best decisions you can on your children's behalf, do what you can to help their immune systems blossom (there's a lot that you can do!) and then be at peace. Worry is a prayer for what you don't want.

RESOURCES

Vaccine Controversies

National Vaccine Information Center (NVIC)
http://www.909shot.com
Publish and carry a number of helpful publications; referrals to lawyers; they also have a free e-newsletter which you can sign up for through their website; very informative website.

Think Twice Global Vaccine Institute
http://www.thinktwice.com
Publishes materials on the vaccine controversy by Neil Miller.

The Vaccine Book, 2nd Edition, by Robert Sears
http://www.askdrsears.com
Current topics on the website include articles on: 12 childhood vaccines, vaccine-preventable diseases, boosting your child's immune system, frequently asked questions, parents who choose not to vaccinate, current outbreaks and epidemics, a vaccine discussion forum, updates and corrections to "The Vaccine Book," Sears' response to criticism of the book, and finding a vaccine-friendly doctor near you.

Dr. Sherri J. Tenpenny
http://www.nmaseminars.com
Informative website, critical of vaccines. Sells DVDs with presentations by Dr. Tenpenny on vaccine topics, including: *Vaccines—The Risks, The Benefits, The Choices—A Resource Guide for Parents,* 2nd Edition

(2005) and *Vaccines: What CDC Documents and Science Reveal* (2003).

For Further Reading

- Gunn, Trevor. *Comparing Natural Immunity with Vaccination.* Worthing, West Suffix: The Informed Parent Publications, 2005.
- Mendelsohn, Robert. *How to Raise a Healthy Child In Spite of Your Doctor.* New York, NY: Ballantine Books, 1984. This consumer approach to children's health care should be required reading for all parents. A chapter on vaccines provides a brief introduction to the subject.
- Miller, Neil. *Immunization Theory vs. Reality: Expose on Vaccinations.* Santa Fe, NM: New Atlantean Press, 1996.
- Miller, Neil. *Vaccines: Are They Really Safe and Effective?* Revised Edition. Santa Fe, NM: New Atlantean Press, 2008.
- Miller, Neil. *Vaccines, Autism and Childhood Disorders: Crucial Data That Could Save Your Child's Life.* Santa Fe, NM: New Atlantean Press, 2003.
- Miller, Neil. *Vaccine Safety Manual: For Concerned Families and Health Practitioners,* 2nd Edition. Santa Fe, NM: New Atlantean Press, 2009.
- Moskowitz, Richard. *The Case Against Immunization.* Alexandria, VA: The National Center for Homeopathy, 1983. This booklet eloquently articulates concerns about possible long-term effects of vaccinations on the immune system.

- Wootan, George and Verney, Sarah. *Taking Charge of Your Child's Health: A Guide to Recognizing Symptoms and Treating Minor Illnesses at Home.* New York, NY: Crown Publishers, Inc., 1992. A good reference book to have on hand for when kids get sick; includes a discussion of vaccines and recommendations which include a mix of vaccinating and (mostly) not vaccinating children. Interesting discussion of tetanus.

Natural Approaches to Developing the Immune System

- Begley, Sharon. "The End of Antibiotics," *Newsweek* (March 28, 1994). The widespread failure of antibiotics hits the mainstream media.
- Brennan, Patty. *Whole Family Recipes—For the Childbearing Year & Beyond.* Ann Arbor, MI: Center for the Childbearing Year, 2007. Contains helpful essays and nutritional hints along with yummy recipes.
- Chuen, Lam Kam. *The Way of Energy: Mastering the Chinese Art of Internal Strength with Chi Kung Exercise.* New York, NY: Simon & Schuster Inc., 1991.
- Fallon, Nancy. *Nourishing Traditions—The Cookbook that Challenges Politically Correct Nutrition and the Diet Dictocrats.* 2nd Revised Edition. Washington DC: New Trends Publishing, 2001.
- Galland, Leo. *Superimmunity for Kids: What to Feed Your Children to Keep Them Healthy Now—and Prevent Disease in Their Future.*

New York, NY: Dell Publishing, 1988. Special emphasis is placed on essential fatty acids and the central role they play in a healthy diet.

- Lappe, Marc. *When Antibiotics FAIL: Restoring the Ecology of the Body.* Berkeley, CA: North Atlantic Books, 1986.

- Schmidt, Michael. *Childhood Ear Infections.* Berkeley, CA: North Atlantic Books, 1990. Describes alternatives to drugs and surgery.

- Zand, Janet, et al. *Smart Medicine for a Healthier Child: A Practical A-Z Reference to Natural and Conventional Treatments for Infants and Children.* Garden City Park, NY: Avery Publishing Group, 1994. Good all-round reference book on children's health.

Homeopathy

Information in the homeopathic section is adapted from the sources listed below. Books with an * were primary sources.

- Birch, Kate. *Vaccine Free Prevention and Treatment of Infectious Contagious Diseases with Homeopathy: A Manual for Practitioners and Consumers.* Victoria, British Columbia: Trafford Publishing, 2007. Provides an introduction to homeopathic philosophy, discusses the side-effects of vaccines, and succinctly outlines the homeopathic prevention and treatment of childhood illnesses.

- Boericke, William. *Materia Medica With Repertory.* Philadelphia, PA: Boericke & Tafel, Inc., 1927. Essential purchase for anyone interested in using homeopathy in the home.

- Curtis, Susan. *A Handbook of Homoeopathic Alternatives to Immunisation.* London: Winter Press, 1994.*
- Head, Christina J. *An Educated Decision: One Approach to the Vaccination Problem Using Homeopathy,* 2nd Edition. London, England: Lavender Hill Publishing Co., 1999.
- Morrison, Roger. *Desktop Guide to Keynotes and Confirmatory Symptoms.* Albany, CA: Hahnemann Clinic Publishing, 1993.
- Nauman, Eileen. *Homeopathy for Epidemics.* Flagstaff, AZ: Light Technology Publishing, 2004.
- Panos, Maesimund, and Heimlich, Jane. *Homeopathic Medicine At Home.* New York, NY: G.P. Putnam's Sons, 1980. Good overall beginner's book, covers introductory materials and remedies for common first-aid crises and acute illnesses.
- Shepherd, Dorothy. *Homoeopathy in Epidemic Diseases.* Saffrom Walden, Essex: The C.W. Daniel Company Limited, 1967.*
- Shepherd, Dorothy. *Homoeopathy for the First Aider.* Saffrom Walden, Essex: The C.W. Daniel Company Limited, 1945. Excellent information on homeopathic wound care and the prevention of tetanus, based on the author's clinical experience treating bombing victims in England during World War II.*
- Starre, Jeffrey. *Vaccine Free Prevention & Treatment With Homeopathy: Alternatives for Domestic & Foreign Disease.* Jewett, OH: Two Hearts Medical Publishing, 1999.*

- Wright-Hubbard, Elizabeth. *A Brief Study Course in Homeopathy.* St. Louis, MO: Formur, Inc., 1977. Good summary of homeopathic casetaking.

Additional Resources
- Homeopathic Educational Services, https://www.homeopathic.com/. Sells books and home remedy kits.
- National Center for Homeopathy, http://www.homeopathycenter.org/find-homeopath. Publishes national directory of licensed homeopathic practitioners; look for an MD who practices *classical homeopathy.*

World Travel

Addressing the issue of vaccines for world travelers is beyond the scope of this book. However, I have come across some resources for those in need that might prove a helpful place to start your investigation.

- To obtain information about specific diseases in other countries, go to http://www.cdc.gov/travel/diseases; vaccination recommendations vary from year to year.
- Dr. Sears discusses whether or not travel presents an enhanced risk of exposure for each disease. In addition, he provides a brief summary of the yellow fever, typhoid, and Japanese encephalitis vaccines. If vaccines are chosen, they should begin at least three months prior to traveling in order to get adequate protection.
- Neil Miller's *Vaccine Safety Manual,* 2nd Edition (2009), discusses a number of vaccines not

discussed here, including most common travel vaccines.

- Another good resource for world travelers is Colin Lessell's *The World Travellers' Manual of Homoeopathy* (Saffron Waldon: The CW Daniel Company Limited, 2004). This book contains a detailed chapter on vaccination and prevention, as well as treatment suggestions for a wide variety of other health concerns when traveling.

Vaccines & Informed Choice

ABOUT THE AUTHOR

Patty Brennan is CEO of the Center for the Childbearing Year LLC, Michigan's premier doula training and childbirth preparation center, established in 1998. She has been professionally involved with childbirth and holistic health care for 35 years as a childbirth educator, doula, doula trainer and homebirth midwife. Patty has served on the faculties of both Washtenaw Community College and Schoolcraft College as an instructor of homeopathy and has been published in the *Journal of Nurse Midwifery, Midwifery Today, The International Doula,* and many other publications. http://www.center4cby.com

Professional Trainings
DONA International Birth Doula Workshops
DONA International Postpartum Doula Workshops
Doula Business Development

Classes for Parents ~ Online Programs Available
Holistic Childbirth Preparation
Breastfeeding & Newborn Care Basics
Introduction to Homeopathy for Family Health Care

Other Books by Patty Brennan
- *The Doula Business Guide, 2nd Edition* (2014)
- *Guide to Homeopathic Remedies for the Birth Bag, 5th Edition* (2014)
- *Whole Family Recipes* (2007)

To Order Copies of *Vaccines & Informed Choice*
Visit our website at http://www.center4cby.com.
Wholesale discount available.

CPSIA information can be obtained
at www.ICGtesting.com
Printed in the USA
LVHW082204260619
622495LV00033B/471/P

9 781512 064094